Suzanne Somers'
EAT, CHEAT, AND MELT THE FAT AWAY

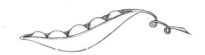

ALSO BY SUZANNE SOMERS

Keeping Secrets

Touch Me

Wednesday's Children

Suzanne Somers' Eat Great, Lose Weight

After the Fall

Suzanne Somers' Get Skinny on Fabulous Food

365 Ways to Change Your Life

Suzanne Somers'
EAT, CHEAT, AND MELT THE FAT AWAY

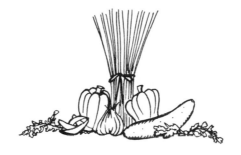

BY SUZANNE SOMERS

Illustrations by Leslie Hamel

Foreword by Diana Schwarzbein, M.D.

THREE RIVERS PRESS · NEW YORK

Copyright © 2001 by Suzanne Somers

Foreword copyright © 2001 by Diana Schwarzbein

Insert photographs and photographs on pages x, 127, 141, 145, 159, 169, 181, 189, 209, 217, 227, and 249 copyright © Jeff Katz

Published by Three Rivers Press, New York, New York. Member of the Crown Publishing Group, a division of Random House, Inc. www.randomhouse.com

Originally published in hardcover by Crown Publishers, a division of Random House, Inc., in 2001.

THREE RIVERS PRESS is a registered trademark and the Three Rivers Press colophon is a trademark of Random House, Inc.

Printed in the United States of America

Design by Debbie Glasserman and Lauren Dong.

Library of Congress Cataloging-in-Publication Data
Somers, Suzanne
Suzanne Somers' eat, cheat, and melt the fat away / Suzanne Somers.
Includes bibliographical references and index.
1. Reducing diets. 2. Food combining. I. Title: Eat, cheat, and melt the fat away. II. Title.
RM222.2.S6549   2001
613.2'5—dc21
00-065605

ISBN 1-4000-4706-4

10 9 8 7 6 5 4 3 2 1

First Paperback Edition

To Al,
My Pal, My Lover, My Partner, My Best Friend,
My Darling Husband

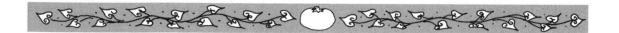

Acknowledgments

I have assembled a great team over the years to assist me with these books. Without them I would be a lunatic, trying to get everything done.

Dr. Diana Schwarzbein has had a tremendous impact on the entire Somersize program. She is the person I turn to for the most cutting-edge information on health issues and hormonal balance through proper eating. I have the utmost respect, gratitude, and admiration for the work she is doing and the help she has so freely given to me. Thank you, Diana.

My daughter-in-law, Caroline Somers, is a vitally important component in the Somersize program. Caroline is incredibly bright and talented. Through her hard work and research she keeps the program up to date by staying on top of the latest medical breakthroughs. But she is so much more to the program than that. She concocts and tests many of the recipes; her input is evident on every page, and she cares deeply about the program. We are very close as mother-in-law and daughter-in-law, but working with her on these books has been a beautiful and rewarding experience and has connected us in a way that goes beyond anything I ever could have hoped for. I love you, Caroline.

My darling stepdaughter, Leslie Hamel, has once again put her unique stamp on this book with her witty and charming illustrations. Her literal way of interpreting the recipes cracks me up. She does this work for me while she is in the midst of her thriving handbag business, designing couture clothing for Hollywood "glitterati," and overseeing and designing my lounge and sportswear line on the Home Shopping Network. I love you, Leslie.

My agent, Al Lowman, is a dream. His input goes way beyond normal agenting. He pores over every page and calls with comments and encouragement. He is supportive and smart. When he has an idea, I really listen because I know his agenda is always to make this a better book. This is the fifth book we have done together, and I look forward to a lifetime of putting out quality books with him. Thank you, Al, for being the best.

My editor, Kristin Kiser, is perfect. She bugs me (in a nice way) to get the project in on time and has no qualms about rolling up her sleeves and going to work when it is needed. I hate doing things like bibliographies, indexing recipes, alphabetizing, and general structure. Kristin and I have done so many books together, she now knows my strengths and weaknesses and picks up the slack in those areas. It's great working with you, Kristin. You're the best!

My husband, Alan Hamel, is a large force in the Somersize program. He is my unsung hero. Supportive, loving, and so damn smart. He sees, as always, the big picture, and is a great visionary. Somersizing has found its way into millions of homes, improving the lives of those who follow the program. I just keep plugging along, writing my little heart out, while he is on the phone, in meetings, and deep in thought, continuously working on making Somersizing more than I ever dreamed it could be. I love you with all my heart, Alan.

My dream team at Crown: Chip Gibson, Andy Martin, Steve Ross, and Wendy Schuman. They are all incredibly supportive, enthusiastic, and the most fun group in all of New York publishing.

A big thanks to my lawyer, Marc Chamlin. This is our fifth book together, and I appreciate your talents.

And to Jeff Katz, my favorite photographer, thank you for your excellence. Jeff

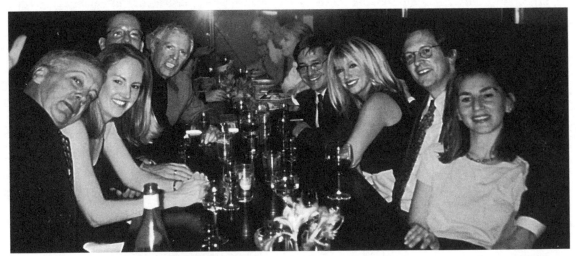

My Dream Team: Al Lowman, Kristin Kiser, Steve Ross, my husband, Alan Hamel, Chip Gibson, me, Andy Martin, and Wendy Schuman, celebrating and enjoying our Number One status with Get Skinny on Fabulous Food.

goes way beyond the parameters of photographer. He comes to the table with wonderful ideas, locations, lenses, commitment, and enthusiasm. It is no wonder that year after year (about twelve at this writing), he is always my first and best choice. Thank you, Jeff. You are a doll!

And thanks to Jeff's team, Victor Boghossian, Jack Coyier, Eddie Chung, and Andy Strauss. You are all the greatest.

Sue Balmforth styled the photo setups, taking those things that are mine and using them in the most unique ways and then adding from her personal treasure trove and from her store Bountiful in Venice, California. If you ever want to find that incredible piece that has eluded you in your travels or your antiquing, it would be worth your while to look up Sue. She is the best and has the world's greatest eye. Thank you for making these photos so beautiful. They "sing," as they say. A big thank you to Sue's assistants, Johnny Ticehurst and Michael Longoria.

Brian Wark did all the floral pieces for the shoot. He has an impeccable eye, always knows the perfect flower to complement the picture. Brian, I trust you implicitly.

Donna Glennon has been with me since 1987. She was the original food stylist on my talk show, *The Suzanne Somers Show*. When I saw how talented she was, I made it a point to keep her with me. Donna and her team prepared and styled all the photos of the food, which look so delicious they jump off the page and beg to be eaten. Thank you to Donna's team Denise Vivaldo, Andy Sheen-Torner, Chris Dinan, Dana Barkdoll, Blake MacHamer, Elizabeth MacDougall,

and Donald King. You are the greatest.

And a special thanks to Debra Murray for creating so many wonderful Somersize recipes for me on Home Shopping Network. You are an inspiring Somersizer and a dear friend.

Thank you to Samantha Deegan for your excellence. Samantha is my personal stylist. When I am in the middle of a food photo shoot, I cannot be bothered by how I look, and it is Sam who is dressing me, futzing, pulling, tugging, making sure everything is just right, while I am standing there saying, "Put more blueberries on the Baked Alaska." Thanks, Sam. You know how much I appreciate you.

Shannon Frost did my hair and makeup; and as with Samantha, I am not easy to pin down on a food shoot. Shannon has to be applying makeup while I am standing over a pot of turkey broth or whatever is on the stove at the moment. But, somehow she always does it. I love the way you make me look. Thank you.

Mary Schuck, thank you for your beautiful cover design. The Somersize books have a real look, thanks to you, and I love the way they are presented. Thank you also to Lauren Dong, Jean Lynch, Amy Boorstein, and Jane Searle—without you all, I know there wouldn't even be a book! Thanks for all your hard work on the production end.

And a big thank you to the girls in my office, Anka Brazzell, Liz Kozakowski, and, of course, Marsha Yanchuck. Marsha has been with us for over twenty years, and we love her like one of the family. Marsha also waded through all the wonderful testimonials and helped me whittle the list down to

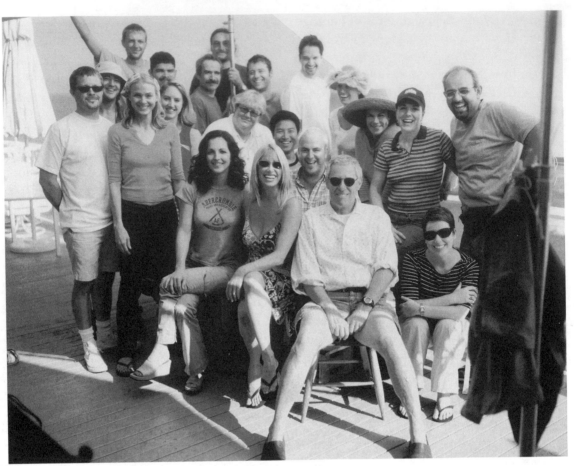

The photo team.

an entire book of testimonials. Your stories also inspire others to take the plunge and start Somersizing; and we know it changes lives.

I have been deeply moved by all the comments I have received on Home Shopping from all of you, and those who call in with your amazing Somersizing results. Likewise, thank you to all of you who hug me on the street and show me your amazing results. I love you and am thrilled with your success.

Thank you to everyone who has helped me bring this incredible program to the public, and thank you to all of you who have achieved such amazing results. I wish you continued success and great eating with *Eat, Cheat, and Melt the Fat Away.*

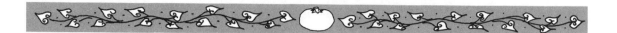

Contents

Foreword by Diana Schwarzbein, M.D. • xiii

Introduction • 1

Part One—Change the Way You Think, Forever, About Dieting and Eating • 5

One   Calorie Counting: Count Your Way Down, Then Back Up the Scale • 7

Two   Standing Out in the Crowd • 14

Three   Sugar: The Sweet and Sorry Truth • 20

Four   Fat: Freeing the Wrongly Accused • 26

Five   Yes, It Works. Yes, It's Safe. • 36

Six   Food Combining: Fact or Fad? • 46

Seven   Hormonal Balance • 53

Eight   Somersizing for Children • 60

Nine   Taking Control of Your Life • 68

Ten   The Program • 72

Eleven   Level One • 83

Twelve   Level Two: Or As I Call It . . . "Cheating" • 103

Thirteen   Frequently Asked Somersize Questions • 115

Part Two—The Somersize Recipes • 125

Appendix • 265

Reference Guide • 267

Bibliography • 271

Index • 273

Foreword

I started studying how the body works when I was in eighth grade. I was twelve years old, having skipped a grade, and I thought that the process of eating something and then breaking it down into smaller molecules was the most fascinating subject in the world. I did not realize at the time that most eighth-graders did not have the same interest in the digestive system that I did.

I continued studying the digestive tract and that led me to the field of nutrition. I started reading every lay book available on the subject since the textbooks were too "dry" to digest. I learned early on what was being taught at that time, which was that foods were categorized into six different food groups:

1. meat, fish, and poultry
2. oils and fats
3. dairy, which included eggs
4. vegetables, both starchy and non-starchy, and fruits
5. pastas, cereals, and grains
6. sweets and desserts

And in order to stay healthy, you needed to eat foods from all of these different food groups.

From the above, I figured I was eating a balanced diet because for breakfast I would have oatmeal with whole milk, a banana, and a lot of added white sugar. At lunch I ate white bread with tuna and mayonnaise. My vegetables would be carrot sticks. For snacks I ate cookies, ice cream, pixie sticks, and cotton candy. At dinner I would have steak and corn on the cob or pasta with butter and Parmesan cheese, if I ate at all. All day long I would drink whole milk and I had on average one regular caffeinated soda a day. I figured that throughout the day I was targeting all the food groups. It may seem naïve now, but since vegetables and fruits were in the same category, I felt that as long as I ate my banana, corn on the cob, and carrot sticks, I was balanced in this group as well.

So, when I developed asthma and irritable bowl syndrome (IBS) as well as a weight problem at age seventeen, it never occurred to me that I had "created" these illnesses from being malnourished. However, I did realize that I was probably eating more refined sugar than was healthy, so I decided to try to eat less sugar and more vegetables, proteins, and fats. I was astonished when my asthma and IBS went away. And was even more astonished to realize that I personally needed to eat more fat in order to lose weight!

When I told my gastroenterologist, the intestinal expert, that my IBS was gone, he said I had outgrown it. When I told my pulmonologist, the lung specialist, that my asthma was "cured," he said that I had outgrown it too! I thought, how do you outgrow a genetic problem? I was being told by these doctors, both subspecialists in their field of study, that I had outgrown a genetic disease and that changing my eating habits had nothing to do with my getting healthy. I knew they were wrong—not only was I healthier, but I had also shed some unwanted pounds because I was eating differently.

These changes didn't happen overnight. I was addicted to sugar and would not have been able to give it up completely cold turkey, and my poor eating habits had led to severe hormonal imbalances that needed to heal before I could be healthy. It took me seven years to heal, but I did eventually heal completely! It took me so long because I had to struggle to learn how to eat correctly. Even more important, I did not have enough guidance on the types of changes I was trying to achieve. After all, it was the late seventies and early eighties, and the prevailing advice was to eat less fat, not more fat! So, my eating habits took several detours as I tried to process what worked best for me.

As a result of my early interest in the digestive system, and my own health issues, I became further interested in studying nutrition. If there is ever any hope of truly understanding nutrition, you need to understand biochemistry, so I threw myself into studying that as well. Since I found both of these subjects to be incredibly fascinating, I decided that I should become a physician and learn more about the physiology of the human body.

Well, it turned out that I was wrong about medical training. Instead of understanding further how the body functions, I was sidetracked into learning how to treat patients with drugs that treat the symptoms, but rarely go to the root of the problem. I was being trained in the pharmacology of drugs instead of learning about normal human physiology.

The truth is that anyone who is ill does not have a normal physiology. They have an altered physiological state that has either led to illness or has been further altered by illness. That being said, instead of learning how to preserve a normal physiology, I was being taught how to treat the symptoms of abnormal physiological states by prescribing drugs. Now don't get me wrong. If you end up in the hospital with a heart attack, I will be the first to give you potentially lifesaving drugs. However, what I wanted to learn was how to prevent that heart attack naturally, without drugs, not what to do once you are in the throes of cardiac arrest.

In medical school, I was bogged down with so much new information about drugs, that I didn't get around to learning much about normal bodily functions. It was not until I decided to further my education and become an endocrinologist (one who studies the hormone systems of the body) that I realized the importance of hormones and their relationship to health and body composition. This was during my eighth and ninth years of medical training!

Deciding to study endocrinology changed my life, as I was finally able to learn in great detail about the importance of hormones and the vital role they play in keeping us fit and healthy. Through hormone study I was able to see how all of our systems function together and how many medical complaints are really interrelated. If you can first identify the hormone system out of balance, then treat the imbalance by either increasing the body's production of the low hormone or giving back the missing hormone (hormone replacement therapy, or HRT), or by lowering the production of a hormone that the body is making in excess, the patient's complaints will *all* go away. It really is miraculous!

Since all hormones play a role in every cell, any hormone out of balance will create multiple varied system problems, which will manifest as multiple complaints. For example: if a person is low in thyroid hormones, or what is known as hypothy-

roid, they are unable to make enough thyroid hormones to keep them in balance. Because this hormone is missing, they can start experiencing a myriad of problems such as hair loss, brittle dry hair, thinning hair, eye dryness, decreased memory and concentration, depression, fatigue, blurry vision, dry skin, weight gain, puffiness, constipation, cold intolerance, swollen tongue, dry mouth, abnormal menstrual bleeding, intestinal bloating and irritability and much, much more. Besides the symptoms above, a patient with hypothyroidism can present, on physical and chemical exam, with high blood pressure, abnormal cholesterol levels, or even Type II diabetes. As you can see, a lot of systems are not working properly when thyroid levels are low. This is because all hormones communicate with all other hormones and if one is missing they are all out of balance.

A lot of different hormonal imbalances can lead to the same type of complaints I just listed. For instance, high insulin levels can cause a lot of the same symptoms as low thyroid hormone production can. This is because low thyroid production leads to, but is not the only cause of, high insulin levels. And vice versa, high insulin levels can decrease the production of thyroid hormones. Since all hormones communicate chemically with all other hormones, all other hormone systems will be altered and the endpoints, which are the symptoms one experiences, will always overlap. Figuring out which hormone system started the cascade of hormone imbalances is the key. In this example, did a problem with the thyroid gland lead to an overproduction of insulin or did an overproduction of insulin, due to a high-carbohydrate, low-fat diet for example, lead to a decreased production of thyroid hormone? If left untreated the cycle of high insulin, low thyroid or low thyroid, high insulin would only worsen.

When the problem occurs because a gland is not functioning well, again as in the example of low thyroid production, then all the person needs to do is replace the missing thyroid hormones with thyroid hormone pills. After six weeks of thyroid hormone replacement, the patient, as long as he/she has only one hormone deficiency, will come back to me now believing that I walk on water! All the multi-system complaints will be "cured." Replacing the missing hormone with the identical hormone that was missing rebalances the system and reestablishes all hormonal communication. And all the symptoms completely go away.

However, when the hormonal imbalances are due to repetitive poor eating and lifestyle habits, there is no magic pill. This is an "acquired" hormonal imbalance. The good news is that rebalancing hormones from the inside out without having to take hormone pills can still be achieved. This is where you come into the picture. Your age, your genetics, your eating habits, your stresses, your exposure to chemicals including the ones you ingest on a daily basis such as alcohol, caffeine, artificial sugars, fake fats, nicotine, refined sugars and preservatives, as well as your activity and exercise routine all determine your hormone balance or imbalance.

Even though you cannot change your age or your genetics you do have more control over your hormones than you might think.

Ninety percent of hormone balance is due to habits; 10 percent is due to genetics. And since your hormones determine your health, you are in control of your health!

The good news is that if you have already made it past your late teens and you have not been diagnosed with a degenerative disease of aging such as cancer, arthritis, osteoporosis, heart disease, stroke, Type II diabetes, etc., then it is likely you were not born with any "inborn errors" of metabolism. This means that if you can take care of yourself, your hormones, which are connected chemically to each other, will all balance each other out. Unfortunately, the bad news is that even if you were not born with a genetic defect of your metabolism, you can still acquire these same degenerative diseases with poor eating and lifestyle habits, since what you expose your body to on a day to day basis impacts your physiology.

Because these "inborn errors" of metabolism are very, very rare, if you are suffering from a degenerative disease, the most likely culprit is years of poor eating and lifestyle habits, not genetics. Think about it, if your health were only about genetics it would not matter what you did on a daily basis. Smoking, drinking, and eating junk food would not have an impact on health and longevity. And as we all know, these things do have an impact. Therefore, health is more about habits than about genetics.

Since most people are not taught about how the body works, what I have seen in my last 10 years of clinical practice and research is that most hormone imbalances are acquired. Of course, since I am an endocrinologist, I do see patients in my office with "real" hormone problems that can only be fixed with either hormone replacement therapy (HRT) if a hormone is missing, or medication to lower excess hormone production, or surgery to remove a tumor that is making excess hormone or blocking new hormone production.

But I want to stress that acquired hormone imbalances are also very real. The difference is that you do not need medical intervention to heal this type of hormone imbalance. It requires changing your habits, good news indeed. Who wouldn't rather have a reversible hormone defect than an irreversible one?

Most people do not understand this connection between hormone balance and proper eating, and thus suffer from the symptoms of poorly balanced hormones. And as I mentioned above, once one hormone is off, all hormones will be out of balance. However, the good news is that you will not keel over and die the minute you eat something that will disrupt your hormonal balance. Your body is designed to make the best of a "bad" situation. The bad news is that nothing is free and your health will one day catch up with your lifestyle.

THE PROBLEM

Why are unbalanced hormones more of an issue today than ever before? Because we are living long enough now that our lifestyle will eventually determine our health. In the past, we would die young and healthy of infectious diseases. We are now assured of living long enough to fall apart. "Falling

apart" before we die is aging. How you age is determined, ultimately, by your genetics. But how fast you age is determined by your daily habits. I call this alterable part of the aging process "accelerated metabolic aging." If you are genetically programmed to live until you are seventy, you can still die earlier because of "accelerated metabolic aging" if you do not take care of yourself. The kinds of diseases associated with accelerated metabolic aging are cancer, arthritis, osteoporosis, heart disease, stroke, and Type II diabetes—these diseases can often kill us before old age, but these are also diseases we can often prevent by changing our lifestyle.

THE SOLUTION

Where do you go from here? You start by eating a healthy balanced diet. If you do not have any hormonal problems then eating balanced meals will quickly reestablish hormonal harmony. If you do not notice immediate results in your moods, sleep, and energy levels then you are either eating incorrectly for your own personal metabolism, you are stressed, ingest too many chemicals, do not exercise enough or exercise too much, or have a hormonal imbalance that needs to be addressed, such as insulin resistance, menopause, thyroid disease, or a low-serotonin state.

If you start feeling balanced right away, but are not experiencing the weight loss you think that you should, you probably just need to give your body more time to respond. There are definitely fast responders and slow responders. If you are losing weight quickly but do not feel good, again, you are not eating correctly for your own personal metabolism, or stress, activity, and chemicals may be a factor.

After you have reviewed your stresses, eating habits, chemical exposures, and exercise routine and you do not feel that these are causing your symptoms, then you may have a hormone system that is failing. A doctor will be able to tell you if this is the case. If you do have problems, here are some simple guidelines for hormone replacement therapy.

1. Only replace a hormone that is low or missing. You do not have to wait for a hormone to completely go to zero before it is replaced. But if a hormone is low because of poor nutrition and lifestyle habits, it is better to establish better habits than it is to replace the hormone. Hormone replacement therapy will always be second best. And remember, the goal is to achieve balance.

2. Replace the missing hormone with the identical hormone. I will use the example of menopause to illustrate this point. When women go through menopause they lose at least two hormones, estradiol and progesterone. These hormones are made monthly in the body by a developing egg. Menopause occurs as a natural aging process of the ovarian system; women run out of eggs. When the eggs are gone, the sex hormones, estradiol and progesterone, are lower than normal. There is not any lifestyle change that a woman can make in order to get her eggs to produce hormones

again. The egg cells are gone forever. It is appropriate to consider hormone replacement therapy in this situation because the estradiol and progesterone production is not going to return to normal.

So, what is the problem? Instead of giving back estradiol, more women are being prescribed Premarin, which contains about 20 different chemicals, all of them derived from pregnant mare's urine. Premarin does not equal estradiol. Estradiol is known to decrease inflammation whereas equinol is known to increase inflammation. Even though estradiol is an estrogen and Premarin is an "estrogen," they are not the same estrogen. Therefore, they are not the same hormone. Both can help hot flashes and irritability, but only one is something our bodies were designed to have. Premarin is a drug that helps with the symptoms of menopause. Giving the body back estradiol is giving the body back what it used to make.

The same can be said of progesterone vs. medroxyprogesterone acetate. Progesterone is a natural diuretic, medroxyprogesterone acetate increases salt and water retention in the body. Even though each is considered to be a progestogen, they are not the same progestogen. Therefore, they are not the same hormone. Although both can help decrease the risk of uterine cancer from exposure to estrogens, only one was designed in the human body. Medroxyprogesterone acetate is a drug used to counter the drug effects of estrogens. Giving the body back progesterone is giving the body back what it used to make.

You may or may not be aware that there

has never been a chemical invented by man or found in another animal species that benefits mankind more than the chemicals that naturally occur in the human body.

3. Mimic normal physiology when giving hormones back. Again I use menopause as the example. The eggs make estradiol and progesterone in a cyclical fashion. In order to have the same effect after menopause these hormones need to be cycled again. Since progesterone blocks estradiol, a prescription of a low dose of estradiol daily with a much higher dose of progesterone daily, will eventually wipe out the estradiol effect. This completely negates the reason HRT is used to begin with. This is called continuous combined or suppression therapy and it will eventually lead to insulin resistance. If a woman starts off with normal insulin levels it may take years before she realizes the changes to her metabolism from taking HRT in a suppressed way. When the high blood pressure, diabetes, heart attack, cholesterol problems, or strokes occur, she and her doctor may not even associate the problem with suppression therapy. It is important to cycle estradiol and progesterone because that is how your body used to make these hormones. Cycling mimics normal physiology and reestablishes hormonal balance.

4. Tracking hormones. One of the most important things to learn about hormone systems is that they are dynamic. This means your habits determine your hormone needs. Before you required HRT, your own body would internally regulate your hormones according to your habits. For example, caffeinated drinks increase the effect of a hormone called adrenaline. Adrenaline is known to block the action of estradiol. When you would drink caffeine, the estradiol effect would be blocked and your egg would increase the production of estradiol.

This extra hormone production would overcome the blockade and you would not feel a thing. Unfortunately, if you are taking estradiol hormone replacement therapy and you have multiple caffeinated beverages in a day, and each day is different, you may never be balanced. There is no way to change your hormone production because you are on a fixed pill containing a fixed amount of estradiol. It is better to change your poor eating and lifestyle habits to keep your estradiol balanced than it is to keep changing the amount of estradiol in your pill around your poor eating and lifestyle habits. Tracking is accomplished by following how you feel and with hormone blood testing.

I hope, after reading this, that you can see how much control you have over your own health. You don't have to succumb to the diseases of aging. The best place to start is with improving your eating habits. Do not skip meals, and always eat meals that are balanced and consist of real foods. Next work on tapering off stimulants and chemicals such as caffeine and alcohol. With all of your newfound energy, then increase your activity and exercise routine. And last but not least, if you have a hormone deficiency, take real hormone replacement therapy.

Suzanne and I have spent the past few years working together as cocrusaders for healthier eating habits. During this time we have become close friends and have developed a mutual respect for each other and our respective work. As I have gotten to know Suzanne better, what strikes me the most is her never-ending quest to get out good information. In Suzanne's new book, *Eat, Cheat, and Melt the Fat Away,* she shares food tips and recipes that will give your body the materials it needs to make hormones. While her thoughts on food combining are outside the scope of my own research, I've supported Suzanne for years now because she advocates eating healthy real foods and has some of the best recipes I have ever come across. So while you are eating foods that are needed for regeneration you are also getting unbelievably delicious cuisine. Do not miss out on this latest edition of her Somersize series; her recipes will improve your health and well-being beyond your hopes.

Have fun eating fabulous food and getting healthier!

DIANA SCHWARZBEIN, M.D.,
author of *The Schwarzbein Principle*

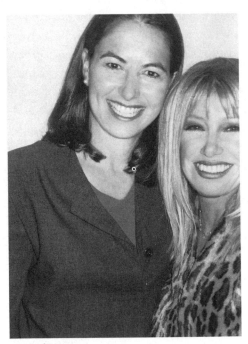

My teacher and dear friend,
Dr. Diana Schwarzbein.

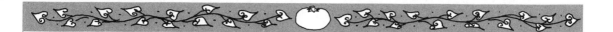

Suzanne Somers'
EAT, CHEAT, AND MELT THE FAT AWAY

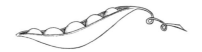

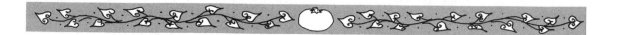

Introduction

It is hard for me to believe how far the idea of Somersizing has come since ten years ago when I learned about a remarkable way of eating while on vacation in France. Our meals were filled with sausages, cheese, beautiful salads, meat, poultry, or fish with divine reduction sauces loaded with butter, plenty of fresh vegetables, and, of course, red wine. But the fun did not end with dinner; for dessert we devoured cheesecake, crème brûlée, and chocolate-covered strawberries. I was shocked to find out this is how the French eat to lose weight! How could that be? Americans had been taught about the dangers of fatty foods: weight gain, high cholesterol, risk of cancer and heart disease. At this rate the French should be overweight and keeling over from heart attacks, yet as a society they eat the richest foods and are still one of the thinnest, with the second-lowest rate of heart disease in the world!

After that revelatory trip, I did some investigating about the French way of eating and found out that unknowingly they practiced food combining, a theory that had been around for over a hundred years. The crux? Keeping proteins and fats separate from carbohydrates, which aids in digestion and weight control. It was considered a controversial theory, because it wasn't backed up by scientific data, yet those who followed the guidelines boasted thin waistlines and better energy. After working with nutritionists and experimenting extensively on my own body, I devised my own food combining program, which finally put me in control of my weight. It was a miracle! It was easy, the food was great, and I lost all the weight I had put on in my forties. I could eat salad with blue cheese dressing, steak with rich brown sauce, vegetables with butter and still lose weight. My hips trimmed down to the size I enjoyed in my twenties. I wanted to tell the world about this amazing new discovery. You don't need to count calories or fat grams or eat prepackaged foods or mix powders or take dangerous pills. I had found the solution—a delicious solution—and I decided to call this weight loss program "Somersizing."

Shortly after I put together my program I wrote the first book in the "Somersize" series, *Eat Great, Lose Weight*. I outlined the program, describing the importance of eliminating sugar and foods high in starch, then combining foods to aid in weight loss and digestion. When I ventured out to promote the book, I came across severe scrutiny, from talk show hosts to medical doctors, questioning the safety of a high-protein diet full of fats. I had read several medical studies that prove *sugar* is actually responsible for high cholesterol and heart disease, but I had a hard time explaining it with my limited medical knowledge. I knew you could eat fat and still lose weight, but I was still uncertain about the role fat played in cholesterol, heart disease, and cancer. For this reason, I kept my fat intake moderate and recommended not to overdo it on the fats in *Eat Great, Lose Weight*. Still, it took some work to convince people that this was an effective way to lose weight because it was so different from the conventional methods of counting calories and fat grams. It took even *more* effort to convince people that this was a safe way to lose weight because we'd been bombarded with scares about eating fat.

Fortunately, word of mouth on *Eat Great* spread quickly and the testimo-nial letters began pouring in, describing amazing success stories of how the weight literally melted away while people ate the most wonderful, forbidden foods of their lives. And to my surprise and delight, people were filling up on fats and their cholesterol was going down! Though I didn't have a medical background, I just knew something big was happening here, and that my early hunch that fat was actually good for you was right.

After the success of *Eat Great*, I received hundreds of letters asking for more recipes. I was planning a follow-up book with a recap of the program and new recipes when fate stepped in and introduced me to the doctor who would fill in the missing "fat gap." Dr. Diana Schwarzbein, one of the country's leading endocrinologists who operates out of Santa Barbara, California, gave me the critical medical information that not only can you eat fat and still lose weight, but also that eating fats is essential to our health! Dr. Schwarzbein is on the cutting edge of medicine and she shared her research with me about the numerous health benefits of fat. She backed up the research I had done on my own about sugar being responsible for weight gain and increased cholesterol, and explained why fats have been given a bad rap. I devoured the information and the second Somersize book, *Get Skinny on Fabulous Food*, emerged soon after.

By the time *Get Skinny* hit the shelves, there was no need to convince anyone of the effectiveness of a low-sugar, high-protein weight loss program. *Get Skinny* sat on the best-seller list with several cohorts nearby. Dr.

Atkins, Sugar Busters, The Zone, Carbohydrate Addict's Diet, Protein Power, even Susan Powter had gone from a virtually no-fat diet to promoting a high-protein plan. Dieters all over the country took their pick from any one of these programs, and most had success in losing the weight. Even with millions of people losing weight, the attacks from the critics continued, lumping all of these programs into one "unsafe" category.

Although there are many similarities among what I advocate and what you'll find in these low-carb plans, I found myself being attacked for elements that didn't even exist in my program! For example, I was asked to appear on a show and a nutritionist was criticizing *Get Skinny* because, she claimed, it is unsafe to eliminate an entire category of food (such as carbohydrates) from one's diet. She obviously had not even read my books and had no idea that my program includes and *promotes* whole-grain carbohydrates for necessary roughage and a great source of energy.

Yes, there are several "diet books" with similar high-protein philosophies to lose weight . . . *BUT MY PROGRAM IS DIFFERENT FROM THE REST!* I was compelled to write this third book, *Eat, Cheat, and Melt the Fat Away,* to show how different Somersizing is from plans like the Atkins diet that eliminate food groups. First of all, my program is *a balanced plan* with all the necessary vitamins and nutrients to keep your body in tip-top shape. Second, Somersizing is a plan for life, *not a crash diet* that will cause you to screw up your metabolism and then gain all the weight back. Third, it's *easy*

to follow—no measuring and no counting calories, fat grams, carbohydrates, or portion sizes. This program is also *backed up by sound medical studies* that will explain why sugar, not fat, is the real enemy. Finally, *my food is by far the tastiest and most delicious,* if I do say so myself. I can't tell you how many people write to me to say that they have never eaten such wonderful food, and they can't believe they're losing weight, too!

I couldn't let people think that Somersizing is just another high-protein, low-carbohydrate plan. With my third book in the Somersize series, you will find ample evidence to change the way you think, forever, about dieting and eating. If you haven't read *Eat Great, Lose Weight* or *Get Skinny on Fabulous Food* and are new to the program, hold on to your hat—better yet, hold on to your pants, because they'll be falling off your new slim waistline in no time. And get ready to eat some of the best food of your life. For those of you who are continuing the program, you will love, love, love, all the new recipes, like Baby Lamb Chops with Parmesan Crusts and Sweet Tomato Sauce, Deep-Fried Turkey with Fried Onions and Herbs, and Buffalo Wings with Blue Cheese Dip—*yum!* I have had such fun creating these delightful meals with sinfully delicious ingredients.

Here's a preview of what you'll find in *Eat, Cheat, and Melt the Fat Away.*

• I'll recap my Somersize program so you can get down to your goal weight and enjoy the slim new you.

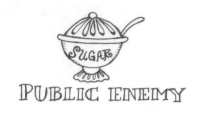

PUBLIC ENEMY

• I'll explain all the high-protein plans on the market, comparing and contrasting so you can see for yourself why Somersizing is the safe, effective, and delicious choice.

• You'll learn why sugar (and hidden sugar found in many foods) is the body's greatest enemy. I'll explain the connection to raised insulin levels and the numerous health risks from such elevated levels. Plus, I'll tell you about a miracle; my new Somer-Sweet, a natural sweet fiber that won't spike insulin levels and is 99.9% chemical free.

• I'll show you medical research that explains the importance of fat in our diets to promote weight loss, and optimum health from the inside out.

• We'll take an overall look at hormonal balance, from childhood to puberty to childbearing years to menopause and see how hormones are the key to our health and well-being.

• I'll answer the most commonly asked questions and concerns about the safety and health benefits of Somersizing in a chapter called "Yes, It Works. Yes, It's Safe."

• In Level Two, or as I call it "cheating," I'll teach you how to "cheat" without completely blowing it. If you never indulge in sweets, you may feel deprived and then go hog wild on a bag of doughnuts and end up going off the program completely. I'll show

you how to incorporate little cheats here and there so you never feel deprived and can still feel proud of your shrinking figure.

• Since many of us overeat to hide from emotional issues, I've devoted a section to dealing with those issues that keep us from living happy and productive lives. You'll learn how to take the focus off the outside things that keep us down and focus on you and what you can actively do to make your life and your body exactly the way you want them to be.

• A chapter that lists some of the most frequently asked questions about Somersizing I've received throughout the years, such as questions about what you can eat and when you can eat it.

• Testimonial letters from people just like you who have committed to this lifestyle and are now savoring the food and savoring the results.

• And of course, new recipes . . . more than 100 of them, including new desserts made with SomerSweet so they are sweet, delicious, chemical-free, and perfect for Level One! All the recipes will tickle your taste buds, delight your family, and leave your guests begging you to host the next party.

Come along, fellow Somersizers. We have a lot to cover, a lot to eat, and a lot to lose!

Part One

CHANGE THE WAY YOU THINK, FOREVER, ABOUT DIETING AND EATING

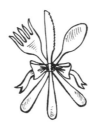

ONE

Calorie Counting: Count Your Way Down, Then Back Up the Scale

How many times have you stood in front of your closet and completely ignored an entire section of clothing? Before I discovered the Somersize solution, I would stand in front of my crammed closet and think to myself, "Someday I'll fit into my skinny clothes again." My clothes spanned three to four sizes, my super-skinny clothes, my normal clothes, my need-to-lose-5-pounds clothes, and my fat clothes. When an important event was pending, I would muster up the willpower to go on a strict diet to get down to that "skinny" outfit.

My diets always consisted of severely cutting down on calories—adhering to minuscule portions of tasteless food. Or I'd eat diet food supplements like shakes or prepackaged food with the consistency of cardboard. I got results, but I suffered! I would lose the weight, but how I missed my dear friend, delicious food! How I missed preparing wonderful meals for myself and my family.

(Well, c'mon, if *I* was going to suffer you don't think I could watch my husband, Alan, indulge around every corner!)

I would get down to my "skinny" clothes for the date I needed to look my best, and then I would go home and reward myself with a feast of all the glorious treats I'd been missing. I'd make roast chicken with gravy, mashed potatoes loaded with butter and cream, and vegetables tossed in butter and Parmesan cheese. And since I hadn't eaten sweets for sooooooo long, I'd bake a sinful chocolate cake and devour two large pieces (plus a few extra forkfuls as I was cleaning the kitchen).

Of course, I would vow to get right back to a "healthy" way of eating so that I would not destroy all the progress I had made. I wouldn't stay on the strict diet, but I would try to eat balanced meals like a "normal" person. Before too long I'd find myself creeping from the skinny clothes into the

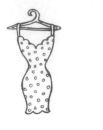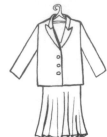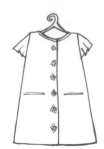

normal clothes. I wasn't eating that much! Why was the weight coming back so fast? When I could no longer squeeze my way into my normal clothes I'd graduate to my need-to-lose-5-pounds clothes. Then I'd either start another diet, or move on into my fat clothes.

The cycle continued, year after passing year. I was never obese, but once I hit forty, I seemed to have a constant battle with my weight, a battle that spanned about 15 pounds. I knew I was to blame. I had no willpower. If only I had the appetite of a bird, then I could always be thin. If only I could resist delectable butter sauces and chocolate brownies. If only I could survive on a starvation diet. If only I could devote three hours a day to exercising. But, no. I was lazy and without conviction, and my fat clothes and I would have to live with the consequences.

Now I realize I could not have been more wrong. *I was not to blame. And neither are you.* Ninety-five percent of us who go on diets gain back all the weight and often more. Why? Are we all just lazy slobs with no willpower? Conventional dieting in the past few decades has presumed that cutting calories and increasing activity level is the key to weight loss. We've all tried it and succeeded for limited periods of time, but *cutting calories is only a temporary weight loss solution.* It is also a potentially dangerous weight loss solution.

SENDING YOUR BODY INTO SURVIVAL INSTINCT

Here's what happens physiologically when you reduce your calorie intake. Let's say your body is used to 1,500 calories a day and you reduce your intake to 1,000 a day. Since your body is used to running on 1,500 calories a day, it must make up for the missing fuel source first by burning off your glycogen and protein stores. (Glycogen is stored with water, and therefore weighs more than fat. The scale may reflect a substantial weight loss due mostly to the loss of water, not fat. That's what the term *water weight* means.) After your glycogen and protein stores have been depleted, then your body will begin to burn off your fat reserves to provide you with enough energy to get you through the day. This initial burning of fuel is why you will lose weight when you cut your calories. After this initial weight loss, many of us reach that frustrating plateau. We're still counting every calorie, yet we've stopped losing weight. Why won't our damn bodies cooperate? *It's survival instinct.* As our glycogen and protein stores are being depleted, our metabolism will actually slow down to keep us from starving to death. Your body adapts to survive on less fuel than it needed before. Plus, your new lower metabolism means

you have a slower-running machine— quite simply, less energy to get through the day, leaving you tired and listless!

Sound familiar? Tired, deprived, and a halt in weight loss. These are all the trappings of a low-calorie diet. But it gets even worse. Your body recognizes that it's not getting enough food, so it starts to store away a portion of the food. It may use, say, 800 calories for fuel and store 200 as fat for later use. So even though you're still living

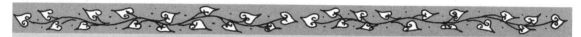

Dear Suzanne,

I wanted to write to you to tell you my story. My story is a little different because for about ten years I starved myself, always wanting to eat but knowing food would make me heavy. I was diagnosed with anorexia and had gone for help but was never able to find the answers for how I could eat right and remain a healthy weight. I gained 30 pounds in the last six years and never thought I could lose this weight the healthy way— until I purchased your book *Get Skinny on Fabulous Food*.

Well, Suzanne, my life is changed forever. I started your way of eating and started feeling so different, so healthy that after the first three weeks I would not weigh myself, fearing I was gaining weight because I could not comprehend eating this much and losing weight. I was shocked on the third week to have lost ten pounds. I have been on this for six months and as of now, I have lost 26 pounds. I am at my goal weight and now I am on Level Two. I can look in the mirror finally after 37

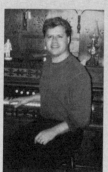

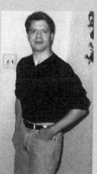

before   *after*

years and honestly say, "You didn't even have to starve, John." The amazing part is that I have lost weight in the right places. Never before have I felt so good about my body. I weigh my perfect weight of 164 pounds and I have been told by others that I look perfect, and for the first time, I feel perfect. I have lost the urge to starve because now I can eat. I have always loved food and now I am able to enjoy food without any guilt.

Sincerely,
John Ziglar

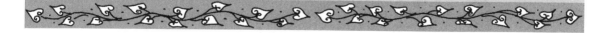

on poached chicken, rice cakes, and celery sticks, you may actually start to gain a couple pounds. That's when the deprivation outweighs the results and we feast on any and every morsel we can get our hands on. It gets worse still. By cutting our calories in the first place, we have forced our bodies to slow down our metabolism, so our body actually needs fewer calories to survive than it did before the diet. When you go back to eating your previously "normal" 1,500 calories a day, your body will have an *excess* of fuel, because it has adapted to survive on 800 calories a day. That leaves 700 calories that could be stored as fat for later use! That's why we gain all the weight back and then a little extra—it's our new lower metabolism, all thanks to cutting back on those calories.

Cutting calories lowers our metabolism and puts our bodies on an unhealthy diet roller coaster with physical and emotional ups and downs that all of us would like to eliminate. Somersizing will help you heal your ailing metabolism. I swear to you, you will never have to diet again. All you need to do is commit to this simple and delicious lifestyle and you will reprogram your metabolism. My closet is no longer stuffed with a spectrum of variously sized clothes. I have my skinny clothes and my skinny clothes and I have Somersizing to thank for it. And guess what? I still eat roast chicken (including the skin!) smothered with mouthwatering gravy. I still cover my vegetables with butter and Parmesan cheese. I still eat salad with real dressing. I just stay away from the potatoes. And occasionally I still treat myself to sinful chocolate cake.

THE SIMPLE WAY TO MELT AWAY

In this book, I'll show you how *you* can eat sinfully rich foods, in abundant portions, in a way that reprograms your metabolism to burn fat and give you a constant source of energy. Level One is the weight loss portion of the program. I'll explain the specifics later on in this book, but here's the basic overview. First I eliminate a small list of foods that wreak havoc on our systems, like sugar, white flour, and potatoes, and then I eat normal everyday foods in combinations that aid in digestion and weight control. In order to increase your metabolism, you must eat food! *I eat whenever I am hungry. I do not skimp on portions. I eat until I am full and I never skip meals.*

Here's how it works. I have taken readily available foods and categorized them into four Somersize groups:

Pro/Fats: Includes proteins like meat, poultry, fish, and eggs, and fats in their natural state like oil, butter, cream, and cheese.

Veggies: Includes a whole host of low-starch, fresh vegetables, from artichokes to peppers to zucchini and more.

Carbos: Includes whole-grain pastas, cereals, breads, beans, and nonfat dairy products.

Fruits: Includes a huge variety of fresh fruits, from apples to peaches to tangerines and more.

The group of foods I eliminate are called Funky Foods, because they don't fit into any of the four Somersize Food Groups.

Funky Foods: Includes sugars, highly starchy foods, caffeine, and alcohol. (You will find complete lists of all of these food groups in the following chapters.)

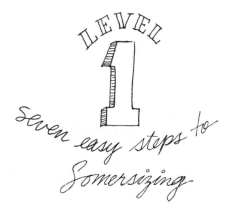

Here are the basic guidelines of Level One, the weight loss portion of my program.

SEVEN EASY STEPS TO SOMERSIZING

1. Eliminate all Funky Foods.
2. Eat Fruits alone, on an empty stomach.
3. Eat Pro/Fats with Veggies.
4. Eat Carbos with Veggies.
5. Keep Pro/Fats separate from Carbos.
6. Wait three hours between meals if switching from a Pro/Fats meal to a Carbos meal, or vice versa.
7. Do not skip meals. Eat at least three meals a day, and eat until you feel satisfied and comfortably full.

Seven easy steps. These seven easy steps are your ticket to freedom. Freedom from the diet roller coaster, and freedom from the extra weight that surrounds the skinny person inside you. As long as you follow all of the Level One guidelines, you may eat until you are full and still lose weight. That's the honest truth. Nowhere in this book will you read that you have to mix powders or take pills or count calories and fat grams, or fast for the first week. Just follow these seven easy steps, enjoy delicious flavorful foods without ever going hungry, and you will reprogram your metabolism to help you lose weight and gain energy.

I know this sounds too good to be true, but millions of Somersizers can't be wrong. They have lost weight and still get to eat all they want every day. Take a look at what you might eat in a sample day if you are Somersizing. You could start your morning with a piece of fruit, then have a shower and follow up with a bowl of whole-grain cereal with nonfat milk. For lunch you might choose a large Caesar salad with chicken and a side of sautéed vegetables sprinkled with Parmesan cheese. In the afternoon you could decide to snack on fresh fruit or a hard-boiled egg. For dinner, try a green salad with blue cheese dressing, a big juicy steak, a side of broccoli . . . covered with cheese sauce if you like and even a bowl of my sugar-free Vanilla Bean Ice Cream made with my miraculous new SomerSweet. No deprivation here.

The magic to losing weight while eating such rich food is correctly combining the foods you eat at every meal. Your perfectly combined steak dinner could be instantly

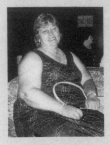

before

Dear Suzanne,

I have been battling being overweight for most of my life, but after the birth of my second child almost 20 years ago, I began to really lose the battle. In that 20 years, I tried various diets, but have always given up after a couple of days. The temptation of chocolate and snacks always won out.

This summer I took a trip to Alaska and when the pictures came back, I got a real wake up call. Since I usually avoid cameras, scales and mirrors, I was surprised that I looked so bad. Not long after that day I saw a show on you. After that show, I went to the library and checked out all of your books. I thought the Somersizing program was worth a try. I knew that I could not get on the scale every morning and counting calories was tedious and unsuccessful. You didn't say I had to do either of these things, just change how I combined foods and give up a few things. I could eat all I wanted of the foods on the program, and that felt good to me.

When school started the last week of August I began Somersizing. I found it pretty easy to follow and my cravings for chocolate and snacks were easier to deny than I could ever remember. Amazingly, by September 8 I could already move my belt over one notch, and I noticed a distinct increase in my energy level. It has been a little more than two months since I started Somersizing. I can't tell you how many pounds I have lost as I am still not using the scale, but I have dropped three pants sizes and one top size. My shoes fit better and I even had to begin wearing my original wedding ring when the larger one I bought several years ago kept falling off! My energy level remains high and I'm not hungry at all.

How can I ever thank you, Suzanne, for sharing this way of life with all of us? I think it is a way of eating that I can live with the rest of my life. My will power comes from the dramatic results I see nearly every week. Although my original goal was just to drop a size or two, I now feel that I may actually be *thin* someday.

Roberta Layton

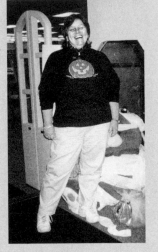

after

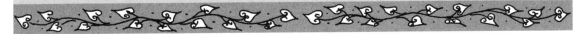

destroyed by eating a potato and a white roll with it, or having a plate of fruit for dessert. Fruit should not be combined with other foods because it causes gas and bloating and may upset the digestive process of other foods. We keep proteins and fats separate from the carbos. But you do enjoy whole-grain carbos on the Somersize plan when eaten at the right times—they are especially great in the morning, with nonfat dairy products. What a perfect energy boost for the beginning of the day!

Change the Way You Think, Forever, About Dieting and Eating

Overall, look at the balance of foods— we eat plenty of fresh fruit and vegetables to provide fiber, vitamins, and minerals; we get whole-grain carbohydrates for energy and additional fiber; and we supply our bodies with the protein and fat from meat and dairy products that is so essential to our

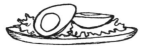

good health. By eating *real* foods instead of processed and refined foods, we are supplying our bodies with the building materials they need to keep us healthy and youthful— not just on the outside, but on the inside as well. There is nothing healthy about replacing real food with fat-free products that look like real food, except for the absence of any nutritional benefit!

When Somersizing, you are eating delicious foods, in combinations that make your digestive system run like clockwork. Food is digested smoothly and efficiently. Your body extracts what it needs and discards the remainder while you melt away pounds and have more energy than ever before. And because it's so easy to eat this way, you can easily dine in just about any restaurant, and you can prepare meals for yourself by using any of my Somersize recipes or creating Somersize favorites of your own. Simple. Effective. Incredible!

Later on, when you reach your goal weight, you will graduate to Level Two, the maintenance portion of the program. We loosen the reins a bit and show you how to Somersize

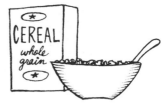

for the rest of your life, without your weight fluctuating more than a couple of pounds.

That's the basic overview of the program. For those of you who did not read my first two books, *Eat Great, Lose Weight,* and *Get Skinny on Fabulous Food,* you are probably still skeptical. I understand. We have been so brainwashed into thinking a low-fat, low-calorie diet is the only way to safely lose weight that any program contrary to that notion sounds like quackery. I promise I will not lead you astray. I have always believed that my program is safe and effective because I gathered information from many doctors and nutritionists while creating it. But this information is on the cutting edge and not universally accepted. Now, because of Dr. Schwarzbein's additional clinical research on sugar and fat, I have more medical research to back it up. Not only is Somersizing safe and effective, it is *essential* to our health. Please don't confuse my program with other high-protein diets that severely restrict certain food groups, like fruit and carbohydrates. Somersizing is a balanced plan that ensures you get all the necessary nutrients and building blocks your body needs in order to thrive. Your body will love it from the inside out.

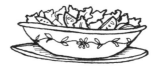

TWO

Standing Out in the Crowd

What do you think of when someone says the word *diet?* Deprivation, measuring, calculating, prepackaged foods, pills, powders, the weight loss roller coaster, which I talked about in the first chapter, are probably the first things that come to mind. This is the reason I do not call Somersizing a diet. Somersizing is really a delicious and enjoyable lifestyle that will help keep you slim and healthy forever. Recently, dieting has taken on new implications with all the high-protein plans out there that offer promising results, but scare the medical community. Well, if you think Somersizing is just another trendy high-protein diet, think again.

As I said in the introduction, I am tired of the critics piling all the high-protein programs into one category as if they all should be disregarded as unsafe. I don't believe that any of the nutritionists or doctors who challenge me have actually *read* my books! They look me right in the face and tell me how unhealthy it is to eliminate all carbohydrates from one's diet. I look over my shoulder, thinking they must be talking to someone else. I do not promote eliminating all carbohydrates . . . quite the contrary. Somersizing includes unlimited low-starch vegetables, fresh fruit (both are made up of carbohydrates), and whole-grain carbohydrates.

Since my program gets compared to so many others on the market, I thought I'd better read these other books so that I could understand the difference, if any, between Somersizing and the others. I also talked to several people who have tried these diets and I collected their feedback on how easy or difficult they were to follow and what kind of results they experienced. Although I found many similarities to Somersizing, there are distinct differences that I feel should be pointed out. Still, I would argue that any one of them is a better choice than a low-calorie, low-fat diet! Take a look at my brief overview of many of the high-protein diets on the market. By comparing them side by side, you can see for yourself why I think Somersizing stands out in the crowd as the easiest, most balanced, most effective, and by far the one with the best food!

Dr. Atkins' Diet Revolution

First of all, let me say that Dr. Atkins is one of the pioneers in this category. I have a great deal of respect for him. He has had the courage to take on the medical establishment and, in doing so, has paved the way for a new way of thinking.

BASIC TENETS
In the Atkins diet you eliminate sugar and high-starch foods. Meals and snacks consist of protein and fat, with limited carbohydrates. Even low-starch vegetables are initially restricted to low quantities (20 grams per day). A sample meal consists of proteins and fats—hamburger patties with cheese, steak, lobster with butter and a small amount of salad or cooked low-starch vegetables. After the first two weeks, you increase carbohydrates by 5 grams (25 grams per day for week three, 30 grams per day for week four, etc.) until you find your "Critical Carbohydrate Level for Losing."

WHY PEOPLE LIKE IT
No counting calories, no counting fat grams. Eat as much as you want of rich, flavorful food like steaks, butter, cheese, and eggs. Very effective for weight loss because

carbohydrates are so restricted. Followers also boast lowered cholesterol levels because the hormone insulin is lowered.

WHY PEOPLE DON'T LIKE IT
You don't have to count calories or fat grams, but you do have to calculate carbohydrates. Even if it's just a cup of lettuce, you have to calculate *any* carbs and make sure not to go over your daily limit. Critics feel the program is not well balanced because a major food group is completely excluded. Others feel a high-protein diet of this kind causes bad breath, body odor, and stress on the kidneys. The most vehement argument is over whether this type of diet will increase your cholesterol and risk of heart disease, although Atkins strongly repudiates these claims with research that raised insulin levels are actually responsible for increased cholesterol. (My research supports the insulin connection as well.)

Protein Power

Written by Dr. Michael Eades and Dr. Mary Dan Eades, this program is a classic high-protein/low-carbohydrate diet similar to the Atkins Diet, but with restrictions on the amount of protein and fat as well as carbohydrate.

BASIC TENETS
Eliminate sugar and high-starch foods. Calculate your lean body mass and percentage of body fat to determine your daily protein requirements. Along with your protein, eat no more than 30 grams of carbohydrates total per day. Add as much fat as you want as

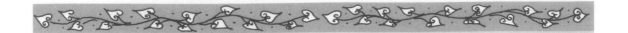

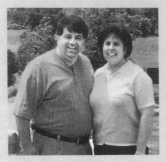

before

Dear Suzanne,

Having attempted numerous diets and weight loss programs over the years—namely everything from "cabbage soup diets" to Weight Watchers—my husband and I were quite skeptical when we first heard about Somersizing and the amazing results that it supposedly yielded. However, this past summer, after I had finished my school year duties as a secretary at our local high school, we decided to give it a wholehearted try. On June 30, 2000, my husband and I embarked on our new journey into a different lifestyle, one that we hoped would finally give us the ongoing positive feedback that we needed.

We immersed ourselves in your program as totally as we possibly could. We ate fruits alone, on an empty stomach, ate proteins/fats with vegetables, ate whole-grain carbohydrates with vegetables and no fat, and most importantly and by far the most difficult to do, eliminated "Funky Foods." We were definitely white bread and potato devotees. We loved French fries and all types of bread. This was by far the hardest part of the program to get used to, but we persevered.

After about three days we had not seen immediate results, and I was craving some potatoes and bread. However, my husband set me straight. He needed to lose weight for health reasons, and so we continued. Summer was the perfect time of the year to Somersize, since we both love salads, and were able to load up on the bounty of summertime vegetables available in New Jersey.

Slowly but surely the weight came off. Combined with daily exercise, the pounds melted away. Soon it became apparent that we were definitely changing our body shape and configuration, because our old clothes were so loose fitting that it was an effort to keep both our shorts and our tops from looking like tents.

The last week of July, my husband scheduled an appointment with our family doctor to make sure that it was OK to be on the plan. Needless to say, since my husband had lost 13 pounds by that time, the doctor was quite impressed and curious as to how he had done it. When he mentioned Somersizing to the doctor, he said he approved of it as a less radical form of the Atkins Diet, and safer too. Just to be on the safe side, my husband had blood work done to verify that his cholesterol readings were all in line with previous tests. The results came back magnificently—total cholesterol went down from 222 to 202, LDL cholesterol went from 160 to 148, and HDL cholesterol went from 35 to 40. Also triglycerides went from 137 all the way down to 72.

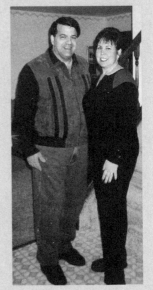

after

This was all the proof that we needed. We stayed on the program for the balance of the summer until I had to go back to my job right before Labor Day. The results: My husband lost 27 pounds, and I lost 18 pounds! We are sticking to the Somersizing diet as much as we can with our busy schedules. But we fully intend to immerse ourselves in the program again next summer, with expectations to lose another 10 to 20 pounds each, all the while enjoying great food that you've given us recipes for. Your program has been a blessing, Suzanne, and we can't thank you enough!

Sincerely,
Sandy and Peter Alexander

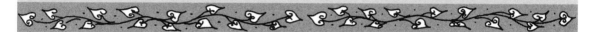

long as you choose from the authors' list of "healthy fats," like olive oil, avocado, and butter.

Why People Like It
Three meals a day plus snacks including rich foods, like meat, cheese, and eggs.

Why People *Don't* Like It
Requires a lot of calculating for everything that goes in your mouth, proteins and carbs alike. Very restrictive on carbohydrates—only 30 grams a day, which is not much. (One slice of whole-grain bread and an apple will put you over 30 grams.)

Carbohydrate Addict's Diet

Dr. Rachel Heller and Dr. Richard Heller identify "carbohydrate addiction" and have created a program to help the addict control the cravings.

Basic Tenets
Eat two restrictive meals a day that consist of only 3–4 ounces of meat, fish, or fowl, 2 cups of vegetables or salad, and 1–2 table-

spoons of fat. For your third meal of the day you get a "Reward Meal," which can be anything you want with no portion limits as long as you eat it within a one-hour time period.

Why People Like It
The Reward Meal allows you to eat whatever you want at least once a day. Some people are willing to suffer for two meals a day to save up for their Reward Meal.

Why People *Don't* Like It
Restrictive fats and portion size make those two restrictive meals a day a real drag. Weight loss is a little slower due to the reward meal.

The Zone

Barry Sears, Ph.D., devised a plan for peak mental and physical performance.

Basic Tenets
Eliminate sugar and high-starch foods. Calculate body fat and lean muscle mass to determine daily protein quotient. Each meal

and snack consists of specific portions of protein, fat, and carbohydrates.

WHY PEOPLE LIKE IT
Well-balanced, nutritious foods in moderate amounts. Increased energy and stamina.

WHY PEOPLE *DON'T* LIKE IT
Technically a little hard to understand. Calculating to get started can be confusing. Tedious measuring and portion control at every meal and snack.

Sugar Busters

Written by three physicians and the CEO of a Fortune 500 company, this program is a low-sugar answer to the problem of obesity.

BASIC TENETS
Eliminate sugar and high-starch foods. For each meal, choose from a list of acceptable foods such as lean meat, poultry, or fish. Add low-starch vegetables or fruit and moderate amounts of whole-grain carbohydrates and fat.

WHY PEOPLE LIKE IT
No measuring. Reasonable portions of foods on the acceptable list, such as lean meats, low-starch fruits and vegetables, whole-grain carbohydrates, and moderate amounts of fat.

WHY PEOPLE *DON'T* LIKE IT
Can't go back for seconds if you're still hungry.

Somersize

Written by lovable ol' me, Suzanne Somers—a regular gal who started getting a little hippy in her forties and was determined to find a way to solve the problem. Contains cutting-edge medical research with a foreword by leading endocrinologist Dr. Diana Schwarzbein.

BASIC TENETS
Eliminate sugar and foods high in starch. At each meal choose either a combination of proteins, fats, and vegetables (i.e., a steak with butter sauce, green beans, and a salad with blue cheese dressing) *or* a meal of whole-grain carbohydrates and vegetables (black bean burrito with whole wheat tortilla and fresh tomato salsa). Eat as much as you want until you are comfortably full. Eat fruit alone, on an empty stomach.

WHY PEOPLE LIKE IT
As with Atkins, you can eat as much rich, flavorful food as you want, but you also get plenty of fruit, fresh vegetables, and whole-grain carbohydrates. There is no fiber shortage here. And the results are miraculous! Somersizers are getting all the essential nutrients to stay healthy while the fat melts off their bodies with minimal effort.

With many of the above programs, you must measure portions and count carbohydrates. When you Somersize, I make it really easy. I eliminate foods high in sugar and starch. Then, I give you four Somersize Food Groups; Proteins/Fats, Vegetables, Carbohydrates, and Fruits. All of the foods in each group are acceptable foods of which you may eat as much as you want. You may eat Proteins and Fats with Vegetables, and you may eat Carbos with Vegetables. You must keep Proteins and Fats separate from Carbos, and you must eat fruit alone. There is no counting of fat grams, protein grams, or carbohydrates. You do not measure portions of any kind. You may eat as much as you want. You may snack as much as you want.

My program is not a trendy high-protein, low-carbohydrate program. Yes, you may eat rich meats, butter sauces, cheese, eggs, and sour cream, but it is also filled with plenty of fruit and vegetables (both contain carbohydrates) and whole-grain carbohydrates. The only carbohydrates I eliminate are those very high in starch. In fact, you may satisfy your carbohydrate cravings at any meal as long as you choose whole-grain carbohydrates.

And people rave about the food! They love the rich, delicious foods and they love the recipes. The recipes are not complicated—even people who say they are not good in the kitchen are having incredible results with this amazing food. They savor the flavor, they savor the results.

WHY PEOPLE DON'T LIKE IT

The only people who don't like it are those who just cannot commit to this or any other eating plan. You must commit to get results.

The main reason that all of these programs work is that they all agree on the major premise that sugar and foods that turn to sugar upon digestion are devastating to the human body. If you learn nothing else from this book I hope you will realize that *calories and fat do not cause weight gain. Hormonal imbalance causes weight gain.* Eating sugar, refined carbohydrates, and highly starchy vegetables causes our bodies to secrete the hormone insulin. When our insulin levels are raised for extended periods of time, our bodies are in a state of hormonal imbalance. This hormonal imbalance leads to weight gain, increased cholesterol, increased risk of heart disease and hypertension, and risk of early death.

The first step in correcting this hormonal imbalance is to eliminate sugars from our diet. It is the key to Somersizing and to our health and well-being. However, many people are confused by sugar. If you think sugar is only found in cakes and candies, read on and you'll realize all the hidden sugars found in many of the foods you eat.

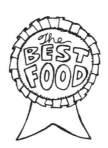

THREE

Sugar: The Sweet and Sorry Truth

I think it's ironic that low-carb diets are so popular these days in the U.S. when we are a country that consumes record amounts of carbohydrates in the form of sugar and sweeteners. Do you know that the average American eats over 150 pounds of sugar and sweeteners (like corn syrup) every year! That's up 28 pounds since the early 1970s! We start our morning off with sugary cereals, Pop-Tarts, or danish. Or we look for low-fat, supposedly healthy alternatives like Nutri-Grain bars, granola, and muffins. Get real! Muffin is cake in a single-serving size! These products are still loaded with sugar and often plenty of chemicals and preservatives.

All my life I have had a sweet tooth. I started baking at a very early age. My mother and I would spend Saturday afternoons in the kitchen baking delicious cakes, pies, or cookies. She taught me how to make the perfect pie crust and how to roll

out tart dough. I remember how the smells filled the kitchen while our treats were in the oven. When the pie came out of the oven and cooled on a wire rack on the counter, I would sneak little pieces off the edge. Oh, the taste. No wonder we call it "comfort food."

These were the seeds of my sugar addiction. For the rest of my life I would crave the sweet stuff. When I was younger I didn't have a problem eating sugar. I could basically eat whatever I wanted and still stay thin. My body had no trouble metabolizing sugar or any other foods. Then I hit forty and suddenly the party was over. I started noticing a thickness in my midsection. My hips were rounder than ever and I had a hard time holding my stomach in. I would eat a meal and then feel bloated and uncomfortable. I tried cutting back on fats. I would carry those little containers of instant noodles so I always had a fat-free snack on hand.

The problem got worse, not better. Little did I know those noodles may have been fat-free, but they were all sugar!

I thought the fat was the problem. I never linked my dips in energy to my sugar intake. I never knew my sugar intake was responsible for my irritability. I never knew my sugar intake was responsible for my rolling hips. And I never knew that eating sugar made me crave even more and more sugar. Then I finally learned that *sugar is the body's greatest enemy!* Surprisingly, sugar is more fattening than fat.

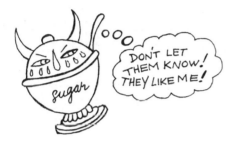

Sugars and starches are carbohydrates. Carbohydrates are one of the body's main sources of fuel. The other is fat. In order to understand why some carbohydrates can cause weight problems, let's look at what happens when you eat carbos. When you eat carbos, they break down into glucose, which causes your blood sugar to rise. When the blood sugar is elevated, it is the job of the pancreas to secrete a hormone called insulin. Insulin balances the blood sugar by carrying the glucose to the cells where it will be burned off for energy. By storing the sugar away in the cells, your blood sugar level becomes balanced. If your cells are filled with sugar and will not accept any more, then the insulin will send the sugar to be stored as fat for later use.

INSULIN—THE FAT-STORING HORMONE

Insulin is called the "fat-storing hormone" because insulin is solely responsible for determining whether food will be burned off as energy or stored as fat. *Insulin must be present for food to be stored as fat.* That is why it is vitally important to identify the foods that cause our bodies to secrete insulin. If we can control our insulin levels, we can control our weight.

As I said, when we eat sugar, our blood sugar is elevated. If our metabolism is working at optimum, our pancreas secretes insulin, which carries the sugar to the cells where it will be burned off as fuel. Here's the hitch. We say people are "insulin resistant" when their cells will not accept any additional sugar. When the cells are closed and do not accept the glucose, the blood sugar level does not decrease, initiating a further release of insulin from the pancreas. This leads to even higher insulin levels and higher blood sugar levels. If the blood sugar is not accepted into the cells to be burned as fuel, it will be converted into fat, where it will be stored for later use. *Therefore, even fat-free carbohydrates, like sugar and white flour, can be converted to fat if we do not need the energy at*

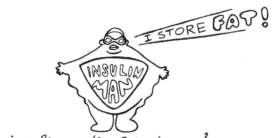

...insulin is the fat storing hormone...

the time we eat. With this information, one can see how the elevation of our blood sugar can lead to weight gain if we eat too many carbohydrates at one time.

Most of us will experience some degree of insulin resistance because it occurs naturally as we get older (explaining why many of us gain weight as we age). Quite simply, as we get older, our metabolic processes slow down and we do not need as many carbohydrates as we did when we were young. But if we don't change our eating habits, those carbohydrates we used to burn off as energy start to get converted to fat and we get thick around the middle as the decades stack up.

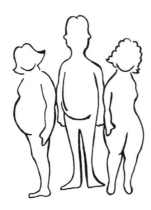

THE TEST—STAND NAKED IN FRONT OF THE MIRROR

Here's the true test, taught to me by Dr. Schwarzbein. Take off your clothes and stand naked in front of the mirror. If you are thick through the middle, then you have a raised insulin level. If you are a man with love handles and a potbelly, then you have raised insulin levels. If you are a woman with thickness around the reproductive areas, such as stomach, hips, thighs, and buttocks, then you have raised insulin levels. If you have raised insulin levels, that means your cells are filling up with sugar and will eventually not accept any more! That means any sugar you eat from that moment on will be stored as fat. When your insulin levels are raised and your cells are filled, sugar in any form (a piece of candy, a bowl of pasta, or a potato) will be converted into fat and stored for later use.

Remember—insulin is a hormone and when we have too much insulin we throw off our body's entire hormonal balance. Hormonal imbalance leads to weight gain, increased cholesterol, and disease. *Stop listening to those who blame fat . . . raised insulin is the proven medical culprit for all of these ills.*

Many of us have varying degrees of insulin resistance leading to weight gain and disease. Even some children have a genetic predisposition to insulin resistance. That's why the crux of this program is to teach you how to keep your pancreas from oversecreting insulin, which will keep your blood sugar and your hormones balanced. With balance comes weight loss. With balance comes lowered cholesterol levels. With balance comes decreased risk of heart disease and cancer. With balance comes longevity. When you heal your insulin resistance, your body will unload the stored up sugar in your cells. That's when The Melt begins. Your body will release all that stored sugar, then it will turn to your fat reserves and break them down to use as an energy source. The result? You get thinner and thinner while your body is being fed a constant source of energy.

WHAT IS SUGAR?

Now that we understand the importance of controlling insulin, let's look at the foods that cause our bodies to secrete insulin. The amount your blood sugar is elevated depends upon the amount and the *type* of sugars you are eating. We must learn what sugars are. Sugar is not only the granulated white stuff you use to sweeten your coffee. Potatoes are sugar. White pasta is sugar. Rice is sugar. Bread is sugar. Alcohol is sugar. Cereal is sugar. Milk is sugar. Fruit is sugar.

However, some sugars cause more of an insulin release than others. Carbohydrates in their refined form are much harder on our systems than those in their natural form. In the last century we have refined most of the nutrients out of our foods. White rice is simply brown rice without the nutty exterior. Brown rice has a wonderful flavor and is loaded with fiber you won't find in white rice. Fiber is essential when we are eating carbohydrates because fiber helps lower insulin levels. And how about white flour? Breads and pastas used to be made with natural whole grains, and as the grains became more refined, we as a society gained more and more weight. We can all improve our health by replacing these processed foods with their whole-grain counterparts.

Some studies show that 75 percent of the average American diet is made up of refined carbohydrates like sugar, white flour, white pasta, and instant potatoes. It's no wonder that obesity is epidemic in our country! And being thin is not just a vanity issue. It is a cause for great concern regarding health.

Obesity is the number two cause of premature death, after cigarette smoking. The statistics are staggering. As a country we are becoming more and more obese, especially since we have adopted the "fat-free" mania that has swept the country over the last decade. These products replace real fats with refined carbohydrates, like sugar and white flour. Here's why the consumption of so many refined carbohydrates is hard on our system.

Complex carbohydrates (like whole grains and vegetables low in starch) cause moderate to minimal increases in your blood sugar, meaning less insulin is released to balance the blood sugar. But simple carbohydrates (like sugar, white flour, and potatoes) cause a sharp increase in blood sugar. This surge of blood sugar gives us a "sugar rush" or a "sugar high." As we now know, when the blood sugar is elevated to such a high level, insulin tries to store the sugar in the cells, but if they become filled with sugar, they will not accept any more. Then the pancreas secretes even more insulin to attempt to balance the blood sugar. This results in an excess amount of insulin in the bloodstream, which causes a condition called "hyperinsulinemia." The higher the insulin levels, the more sugar is converted and stored as fat. (Type II diabetes occurs when the fat cells are also filled, which means the sugar has *nowhere* to go and it remains in the bloodstream.)

It makes me crazy when I see companies promoting fat-free items loaded with sugar and carbohydrates that will make your insulin levels go through the roof. People sit and eat an entire bag of fat-free Entenmann's cookies because they have been led to believe the fat was the only danger. Fat-free cookies are not going to help us lose weight! The fat is not the problem. In fact, it is the sugar and white flour that cause the weight gain! And the chemicals that accompany many fat-free products are harmful to your health. Olestra, the fake fat recently approved by the FDA, must carry a warning label because it adheres to some vitamins and nutrients so that they cannot be absorbed by your body. And it may cause abdominal cramping and loose stool syndrome; so if you really want that bag of fat-free potato chips, you'd better be near a bathroom!

If fat-free cookies, cakes, and potato chips sound too good to be true, it's because they are. Fat has been made the fall guy, but sugar is the body's greatest enemy. Effective marketing has duped our society into thinking if we are eating low fat, we are safely eating food that is healthier for us and will not make us fat. But they don't tell you that *fake food is harmful to your health* and *sugar turns right to fat!*

After this extra insulin has sent the sugar to the fat cells, eventually our blood sugar is lowered to even below its starting point. That's when we feel the letdown or the "sugar low." This sugar low leaves us feeling tired, listless, and artificially hungry. During this time we often feel like taking a nap, or we reach for something sweet or caffeinated to give us more energy—then the vicious cycle repeats. Sugar goes in, blood sugar goes up, pancreas secretes insulin, then blood sugar drops and we feel tired and hungry again, causing us to eat more and

more without ever satisfying our nutritional needs.

Now you are beginning to see the importance of insulin in determining whether the broken-down sugar will be burned as fuel or stored as fat. As I mentioned, some complex carbs cause smaller insulin responses (whole grains, green vegetables) and will usually be burned off from the sugar cells as readily available fuel. Other carbs cause larger insulin responses (sugar, white flour, potatoes) and will often be stored as fat because they contain way more energy than our bodies need for immediate use. A single potato is so high in starch it provides us with more energy than most people need in an entire day. Think about how many excess carbohydrates you eat in a normal day and imagine how much your body actually needs for fuel and how much gets stored as fat. Unless you're a marathon runner, you're probably storing an ample supply of fat reserves from overindulging in the wrong kind of carbohydrates.

You may know people who seem to contradict what I just told you. They live on bad carbs and junk food, wolfing down fries and chips and candy bars and never gaining weight. Keep in mind that each of us is created differently with a unique and ever-changing metabolism. Some people have a perfect metabolism that will always burn the food they eat as fuel—even if it's bad food like refined carbohydrates—rather than storing it as fat. (Other people start out with a perfect metabolism and as they get older their metabolism changes and suddenly they find themselves with a weight problem.) But nothing is free. Even if your friends don't gain weight, they still can be damaged by eating junk food—they are prone to heart attacks, decreased energy, mood swings, and possible early death from poor nutrition.

If you have an imperfect metabolism and want to lose weight or if your weight is fine and you want to achieve maximum health, Somersizing can help you. By eliminating foods that cause large fluctuations in our blood sugar and by properly combining nutritious, delicious foods, we are able to lose weight and gain energy while achieving our maximum health. Most of us do not have a perfect metabolism, but Somersizing can show you how to *get control* over your metabolism. This program can actually heal your ailing metabolism. It's never too late to change.

THE SOMERSIZE SOLUTION

When your body needs energy, it will first look for carbohydrates to burn as fuel. If there are fewer carbohydrate sources available, your body will break down your fat reserves when you need energy. By cutting back on sugar and highly starchy foods, you force your body to melt away your fat reserves as an energy source.

That's the key to Somersizing. We convert our bodies from carbo-burning machines into fat-burning machines. By limiting our sugars and starches, we force our bodies to break down our fat reserves to use as a constant source of energy. No sugar highs and lows—just an even source of energy to get through the day as we watch our fat melt away.

The good news is that you don't have to say good-bye to sugar and starches forever. While you are on the weight loss portion of the program, Level One, the built-up sugar is being emptied from your cells. When you reach your goal weight, you will advance to Level Two, the maintenance portion of Somersizing. In Level Two you may incorporate some sugar and starches back into your eating plans (in moderation). Because your cells are no longer filled with sugar, they can handle moderate amounts without becoming overloaded. That is why on Level Two some previously forbidden sugars and starches are permitted, because they will be burned off rather than stored as fat.

Now with my new SomerSweet, you can even enjoy sweet treats on Level One. SomerSweet, unlike sugar, honey, or molasses, does not spike your insulin. And, unlike aspartame or saccarin, SomerSweet is chemical-free so you may enjoy it freely. Plus, it has no aftertaste. It feels like a miracle to enjoy sweets again on Level One!

So we now are starting to see that sugar, not fat, is the problem. I know it's hard to accept all this information when we live in a society that blames fat for weight gain and poor health. How can we gain control of our metabolism and lose those extra pounds while consuming fat? Let's take a look at this paradox in the next chapter.

Fat: Freeing the Wrongly Accused

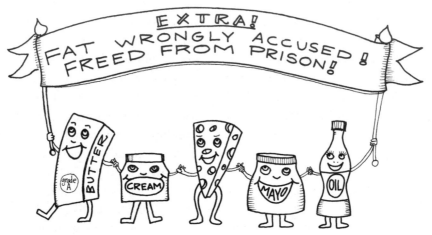

If you've read *Eat Great, Lose Weight* and *Get Skinny on Fabulous Food,* you know there is nothing that makes me angrier than the medical establishment's refusal to see that fat is an important, and necessary, part of our diet. Instead, fat has been portrayed as the primary cause of weight gain, obesity, and poor health. We've all been watching our fat intake so we can lose weight, right? If you just look at the facts, though, you'd see how misguided it is to blame fat for weight gain. In the last two decades Americans have cut their fat intake from 38 percent to 34 percent of their daily calories, and yet in that same time period the average weight per person has increased by 8 pounds! How can

that be? Isn't a reduced-fat diet supposed to help us lose weight? Doesn't less fat in our diets mean less fat on our bodies? Not necessarily. We keep hearing, "Eat less fat. Eat less fat," and we have obeyed. Then why has the percentage of adults who are overweight *increased* by 10 percent since 1980? Over 37 percent of females and 34 percent of males are now overweight. Obesity is rampant in our country, and they say fat is to blame.

As I said earlier, doctors are constantly challenging me about my support for eating fat. They act like I'm telling people to eat a tub of lard with every meal or deep-fry everything! Somersizing is not a license to pig out on greasy chips or oily fries, but a health plan that encourages eating natural fats like cheese, meat, and cream. When you Somersize, yes, you can eat a juicy steak with a mushroom cream sauce. Yes, you can eat chicken with lemon butter sauce. Yes, you can eat taco salad topped with salsa and sour cream. Yes, you can eat tuna salad or egg salad with real mayonnaise.

When you Somersize, you can eat fat and still lose weight.

That's right. Putting fat in your mouth will not add fat to your thighs. Eating dietary fat causes virtually no secretion of insulin, and as we learned in the last chapter, insulin must be present to store fat in the fat cells. Regardless of how much fat you eat, the pancreas will not secrete insulin, *which is the only way fat can be stored as body fat.* As long as you are properly combining, you can eat fat and still lose weight. But you *can* gain weight if you eat proteins or fats *with* carbohydrates. The combination of bread with cheese can be a killer. Here's why.

If you eat a Protein/Fat alone, like a piece of cheese, your body will break it down easily. Pro/Fats will not cause weight gain when eaten alone because they trigger virtually no increase in your blood sugar levels, so there is not a significant insulin response. Pro/Fats can also be eaten in combination with vegetables low in starch (which are also foods that cause little to no insulin production). Therefore, eating Pro/Fats, like eggs, meat, cheese, and butter, will not make you fat when eaten in the suggested Somersize combinations.

But let's say you eat fat *with* a carbohydrate, like cheese with white bread. The body *should* use the carbohydrates in the bread for energy, extract the nutrients from the fat, and discard the remainder. But the carbohydrates in the bread will trigger an insulin response that can lead to both the bread *and* the cheese being sent to the fat cells. So say good-bye to grilled cheese sandwiches on white bread, or baked potatoes with butter and sour cream, or bagels and cream cheese. I know this may sound difficult, but there are so many other foods you can eat in the right combinations, you won't even miss these foods after a while.

Believe it or not, fat is not fattening when eaten alone. You can eat fat with other fats, with proteins or with vegetables in Somersize combinations and still lose weight. And what a pleasure it is to eat this way! I have never felt so indulged on a weight loss program.

Despite my love of fats, I don't want you to think that you should go out and gorge on fat and ignore a balanced eating plan filled with essential nutrients from several food groups.

But I joyfully treat myself to cheese soufflé, butter sauce, or a piece of Brie without guilt. How wonderful not to feel deprived when you're trying to lose weight! I think that's the main reason Somersizing has been so successful with everyone who has tried it.

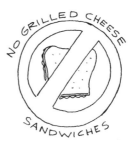

You can incorporate rich, flavorful foods into your diet and still lose all the weight you want; and that helps people stick to the program.

FAT — YOUR FRIEND FOR LIFE

Let's say you understand what I've been saying and you see that eating fat does not lead to weight gain, if you don't eat fat with carbs. But doesn't eating fat increase your cholesterol levels and lead to greater risk of heart disease and even certain types of cancer?

Conventional wisdom tells us that most of those illnesses are blamed on dietary fat. But my research has led me to different conclusions. Actually, insulin resistance is responsible for many of the modern-day maladies, like high cholesterol and heart disease. (Later in this book you can read about the numerous studies that back up these claims.) Eating in proper Somersize combinations lowers insulin levels, which subsequently helps lower your cholesterol, and I've heard it time and time again from all of you who have seen the results for yourself.

When I met Dr. Diana Schwarzbein, I felt like I had met my soul sister in defending fat. Her clinical findings prove not only is fat not dangerous to our health . . . it is essential to our health! If you've read *Get Skinny,* you know I shouted Dr. Schwarz-

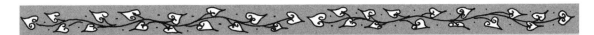

Dear Suzanne,

I had been at my wit's end, trying to find an eating plan that really worked. I had almost totally given up on ever having the figure of my dreams. Then, luckily one day I saw you on Home Shopping Network. I ordered your plan, and after watching the video and absorbing the information in your book, I started working on losing weight.

The diet was so easy, I could hardly believe it! The recipes presented in your book were and are extraordinarily delicious! I was, and still am, not hungry Somersizing. When I cook the many exciting recipes in your first two books, I have meals that are sumptuous enough to entertain my friends.

Somersizing allows me to have a good feeling about what I eat and I do not have to feel guilty when I eat these tasty foods, because I know I will lose weight. I have lost around 120 pounds in one year and two months on this diet. I am a teacher and a graduate student and I stay quite busy, but I do find time to eat my three balanced Somersize meals a day. I can even eat in my favorite restaurants on this plan and eat my favorite foods. I also exercise moderately when I can.

Thanks again for giving us such a great eating plan, and I cannot wait to read your books in the future!

Sincerely,
Rebecca-Rose Lutonsky, MA

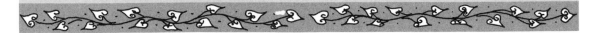

bein's information from the mountaintops. Dr. Schwarzbein explains in her book, *The Schwarzbein Principle,* the important role of fat in creating healthy cells. If we do not eat enough dietary fat we are damaging our cells and our bodies' ability to reproduce new cells. When cell abnormalities develop, disease can set in.

A balanced diet, including fat, is essential to life. When I say fat, I don't mean the fat you give your body in the form of cake, or fat from a candy bar. Even Alan tries to get away with eating bad fat by throwing this in my face! When we drive to our house in the desert we used to stop at McDonald's and treat ourselves to French fries. Since we started Somersizing, this treat has become less and less frequent . . . maybe once or twice a year. That little bad boy in Alan emerges every time he sees a sign for McDonald's. He'll look over at me with that sheepish grin, hoping my willpower will cave. If I don't flinch, he'll say, "Oh, c'mon, Suzanne, we have to get our fat!" Not *that* kind of fat. No one needs that kind of fat.

There are several different types of fat. Some are good, in fact essential to your health and well-being. Others are very dangerous and should be eliminated from your diet. There are two main types of fats: saturated and unsaturated. Saturated fats include butter, lard, coconut oil, and palm oil. These types of fats are usually solid at room temperature. Unsaturated fats are generally liquid at room temperature. These liquid types of fat are categorized as monounsaturated— such as olive oil and nut oil, or polyunsaturated—such as corn oil or safflower oil.

Trans fats are the fats that come from

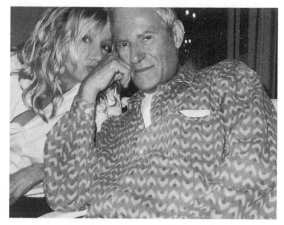

My pal, Al.

polyunsaturated fat, like partially hydrogenated oil. These trans fats are the most dangerous kind because they are completely unnatural. Margarine is an excellent example. We've been led to believe that margarine is a healthier choice than real butter, because butter is saturated and margarine is unsaturated. But margarine is made by taking a vegetable oil and stripping it of its essential fatty acids. The remainder is processed by forcing hydrogen atoms into it. When complete, margarine, which comes in a solid state, is actually more saturated than its original liquid form! Trans fats also occur when we heat polyunsaturated fats (like vegetable oil) for frying. I know it sounds ironic, but you are actually better off frying food in saturated fat—like butter, lard, or palm kernel oil than you are frying it in polyunsaturated oil like corn, safflower, or canola. We've been led to believe these polyunsaturated oils are a healthier choice, but beware of frying foods with them because when heated they become the most dangerous type of fats—trans fats.

In response to the fat scare, many restaurants and food chains boast that they fry only in "cholesterol-free" oils, like canola or safflower. These oils are healthy in their natural state, but become dangerous trans fats when heated to high temperatures for frying! Don't be duped by fat-free propaganda. Eating foods filled with these trans fats is dangerous to our health. If ever I feel weak when Alan suggests we stop for McDonald's French fries, I think about the trans fats in the hydrogenated oil with the combination of potatoes and I am quickly brought to my senses. Trans fats are rampant in the processed foods we eat. It's not just the fries at restaurants. They appear in almost every snack food that comes in a bag or a box at the grocery store—cakes, cookies, crackers, breads, chips, margarine, bottled salad dressings, and more. Many of the low-fat varieties of these foods are filled with trans fats.

And why are trans fats so bad for us? They raise your bad cholesterol (LDL) and lower your good cholesterol (HDL). Plus, they muck up your cells with these fake fats and actually block your body from accepting the good fats it needs to produce healthy cells. Sadly, people are eliminating saturated fats, like eggs, cheese, butter, and red meat, thinking they are the culprit for raised cholesterol and heart disease, when in actuality raised insulin levels and trans fats are the

problem. Since the introduction of fake foods into our society, we have been on a fast road to weight gain and disease. When I was a child my mother baked me cookies made with real butter. That was considered a treat. Now cookies are prepackaged in the grocery store, depleted of any real fats and filled with unhealthful trans fats.

Get back to eating real fats like butter, cream, cheese, sour cream, and eggs! Most doctors will tell you that eating foods high in saturated fats is a recipe for weight gain and a heart attack. They will tell you these are the types of "fatty" foods that will raise our cholesterol. They advise us to stick to unsaturated fats in minimal amounts. So how can I share with you my program with a clean conscience when Somersizing supports eating saturated fats to your heart's content? Because I have done the research and have seen that the majority of the medical community is wrong! Saturated fats are good fats and essential to life. They must be included in our daily meals.

Dr. Atkins, one of the great pioneers in promoting proteins and fats as part of a healthy diet, sites several medical studies that support the notion that the medical establishment is ignoring the evidence concerning the health benefits of fat. There has been an ongoing study in Framingham, Massachusetts, that has followed the diets

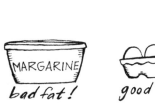
MARGARINE bad fat!

good eggs!

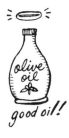
good oil!

THE INCREDIBLE EDIBLE EGG!

Crack 'em, fry 'em, boil 'em, devil 'em, scramble 'em. However you like them . . . enjoy your eggs. So many of us have been told to eliminate eggs from our diets to reduce our risk of cholesterol and heart disease. Nothing could be further from the truth. Eggs are an excellent source of protein and real fat. They have essential omega-3 and omega-6 fatty acids to help produce and re-create healthy cells. Numerous medical studies support eating eggs to lower cholesterol levels! Just make sure you don't eat them with toast or potatoes. Combining eggs with sugars or starches causes the secretion of insulin. With the presence of insulin the eggs and the potatoes and toast could be sent to the fat reserves. Ironically, the raised insulin from the potatoes or toast is what leads to raised cholesterol levels.

I eat eggs several times a week. My mornings often begin with three eggs and I boast perfect cholesterol levels. Even Alan, who previously struggled with high cholesterol, eats eggs several times a week and his levels are now lower than ever! Have no fear of the egg . . . embrace it. It is one of earth's most perfect foods. And please, eat the yolk! The yolk contains the essential fats we need to thrive.

Recently I was having breakfast with my agent, who has adopted Somersizing to lose a little weight. He recited back most of my book, excitedly talking about all the previously forbidden foods he was now enjoying. Then he paused and ordered an egg-white-only omelette, saying he had to watch his cholesterol! It takes some undoing to understand this new way of thinking. Trust me . . . eat the eggs with the yolk *and enjoy the results.*

and health of a large test group of citizens of this city. For many years, this study supported the notion that saturated fats increase our risk of cholesterol. However, recently, Dr. William Castelli, who was the director of the study for many years, has changed his tune. In 1992 he was quoted:

In Framingham, Massachusetts, the more saturated fats one ate, the more cholesterol one ate, the more calories one ate, the lower people's serum cholesterol. . . . We found that the people who ate the most cholesterol, the most saturated fat, ate the most calories, weighed the least and were the most physically active.

That study reminds me of my father. He ate fried eggs and bacon every morning of his life. Everyone told him he was going to die of a heart attack. He lived until the ripe old age of eighty-three—slim as a whistle with cholesterol in normal range. Another study Atkins brought to my attention is a 1997 article in *European Heart Journal,* "The Low Fat/Low Cholesterol Diet Is Ineffective." The authors took a twenty-year look at diets and heart disease and proved that the low-fat/low-cholesterol diet is not effective.

We are on the brink of a turnaround. I can feel it. You still have the die-hard medical conservatives telling us to limit our fat intake and replace real fats with fat substitutes. Others are coming around slowly. They are still adhering to the low-fat diet, but they are recognizing the need to limit sugar consumption. The questions raised by the plummeting health of our low-fat society have inspired several medical studies. More and more data is pouring in supporting the benefits of essential fats. Check out the additional medical studies listed in the back of the book. It's fascinating to read all this research and still hear doctors saying we should limit fats. Get the word out! Everyone should have this critical information.

Real fats are your friend and partner in good health. Your body cannot produce fats on its own, therefore essential fatty acids must come from the food you eat. Let's look at two important essential fatty acids that we must include in our diets to enjoy health and longevity: omega-3 and omega-6. Omega-3 can be found in egg yolks, fish (salmon, tuna, herring, mackerel), nuts, soybeans, canola oil, and flaxseed oil. Omega-6 can be found in egg yolks, dark green leafy vegetables, whole grains, and seeds. (My doctor gives me a supplement called borage oil, which is an excellent source of omega-6, and also helps tremendously to reduce the symptoms of PMS and menstrual cramps.)

These real fats are necessary for healthy cell reproduction. We need fats to make hormones and hormones are essential for breaking down old cells and making new ones. Why is healthy cell reproduction so important, you say? The human body is made up of cells. We must produce healthy cells to thrive. When we deny our body the nutrients it needs for healthy cell reproduction we will start producing abnormal cells. That's when disease sets in. You should care about healthy cells, because if you don't your health is at risk. We must have sufficient hormones to make healthy cells and we must have healthy cells to make more hormones. The health benefit comes from eating *real* fat in its natural state, like butter, oil, cheese, sour cream, eggs, or fat found in meat or fish.

KEEP THOSE CELLS HEALTHY

Dr. Schwarzbein explains that in the normal aging process, hormone levels will decline, causing the subsequent loss of healthy cells. Simply put, aging results when our bodies break down more cells than they build up. Although there is no way to prevent *normal* metabolic aging, our society is on what Dr. Schwarzbein calls a frightening *accelerated* metabolic aging path. Bad eating habits, stress, caffeine, alcohol abuse, and inactivity can lead to extended periods of high-insulin levels, which prematurely ages our bodies on a cellular level. This aging process leads to disease.

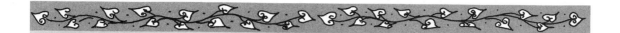

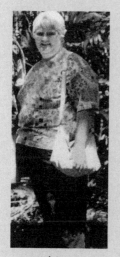

before

Hello Suzanne!

I have to say that I am so thankful I saw you and your hubby on one of the daytime shows. Your hubby mentioned how when you eat the wrong foods he has to leave you alone as it affects you so much. I stopped and listened to what you had to say and then went to the library and checked out your book. I started eating your way November 1 and have lost 35 pounds so far. I feel so good and have much more energy. Between my diabetic husband and me we have had a lot of changes. My husband had gone through colon cancer surgery almost six years ago, and after that he had chemotherapy and radiation. Since then he was having a major gas problem, diarrhea, and eventually acid reflux, all things he had to live with as the doctor said there was nothing to help him. Since eating the Somersize way he has not had a problem with any of them. His diabetes is also controlled. His new doctor asked him if he was really a diabetic as his count is so low. My husband is mostly doing Level Two as he is happy with his weight. My daughter-in-law and son and two children are all now doing the Somersize program. They waited until they saw me lose and get healthy.

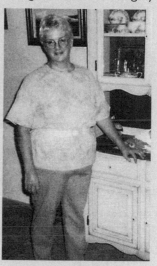

Verna Gamsky

after

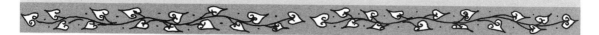

Additionally, when the hormone insulin is present at increased levels, it can disrupt every other hormone system in the body, which can lead not only to excessive body fat, but to degenerative diseases of aging such as different types of cancer, cholesterol abnormalities, coronary artery disease, high blood pressure, osteoporosis, stroke, and Type II diabetes. *Hormone imbalances always lead to disease.* We must control our insulin levels so as not to disrupt every other hormone system in the body!

Furthermore, women who are already going through menopause are at extreme risk of disease. As women age, we naturally become more insulin resistant, which explains why it gets harder to stay slim as we get older. Adopting a high-carb diet exacerbates the problem because all those carbohydrates increase insulin resistance. The elevated amount of insulin in the blood increases testosterone levels, which further blunts the production of the female sex hormones, estrogen and progesterone. Compound the problem with a low-fat diet and you have even less hormone production because we must consume dietary fat to create hormones. Besides the uncomfortable side effects of hot flashes, cramping, and mood swings, an imbalance of these sex hormones means we cannot produce healthy cells! It is at this critical stage that women become vulnerable to disease. I'll discuss later the importance of maintaining hormonal balance in the body for menopausal women, but for now, just remember that eating fat is one of the ways to rebuild hormones.

I hope I've made clear the connection between nutrition and health. Everything we put into our mouths, good or bad, has a direct effect on our health. We all know eating junk food is bad for us, yet I don't think we consider the consequences of the bad food choices we make. Years of poor eating habits cumulatively add up to damaged cells and our bodies' inability to produce new, healthy cells. When we eat poorly, we age faster, not only externally, but internally as well! And this accelerated metabolic aging process leaves us vulnerable to disease at an earlier age. Eating right isn't just about weight loss, but total health that will last us through our lives.

I've explained how important it is to eat real food and real fat to lose weight, but we need to stay away from processed foods and trans fats for another important health reason. Processed foods introduce free radicals

into our systems. Free radicals are molecules that carry an extra electron. Since electrons need to be paired off, these free radicals roam through our system like little home wreckers, trying to steal electrons from healthy cells. This process damages our system on the cellular level. Antioxidants, such as Vitamin E, Vitamin A, and Vitamin C, help to neutralize free radicals. But when we replace real food (which includes natural vitamins) with processed food, we are not supplying our body with the natural antioxidants it needs to fight the free radicals; instead we are introducing more free radicals into our system! The damage that results over time accelerates the metabolic aging process and leads to insulin resistance, then disease, and possible early death. Ironically, two of the most powerful antioxidants, Vitamin A and Vitamin E, are found in foods that contain fat.

Processed foods and trans fats aren't the only things compromising our health. Consider that the average American drinks 42 gallons of sugary soft drinks every year! We are literally killing ourselves with sugar and chemicals that break down our bodies on the cellular level. The sugar and caffeine in one cola wreak havoc on your body by spiking insulin levels. Think about it every time you consider having a can of soda. Imagine the insulin in your body looking unsuccessfully for places to store the abundance of glucose, and visualize how the sugar then gets converted into fat because your cells just cannot accept any more sugar. Visualize the free radicals sweeping through your system, damaging your cells.

With diet drinks you don't have the sugar

to contend with, but you have the additional free radicals from the artificial sweeteners. The most recent studies on the effects of aspartame (NutraSweet, Equal) are frightening. Lab studies have proven irreversible brain damage in laboratory animals. In fact, one can of soda can raise the levels of toxins in the brain of an infant higher than levels that caused brain damage in immature animals. Certainly, no one is filling infants' bottles with diet sodas, but many toddlers drink this poison regularly. And many adults drink diet sodas by the gallon. Since there are not yet any long-term studies showing the effects of aspartame, is it really worth the risk? All for a can of Coke? I think not.

I know I've just thrown a lot of information your way. But try looking at your body the way I look at mine—I visualize all my happy little cells. As I get older I know some of them will die off and there is nothing I can do about that. But I imagine what happens when I am not giving my body the proper combination of nutritious foods, and I see the cells dying off at a rapid rate. When I give my body the protein, fat, and complex carbohydrates it needs, my cells thrive and I feel empowered because I can stave off disease and aging for as long as possible. How wonderful to realize that Somersizing not only keeps me in control of my weight, but also keeps me at my metabolic prime. I know the food I am eating is creating millions of happy cells that keep me young, slim, and healthy.

free radicals..cell damaging culprits!

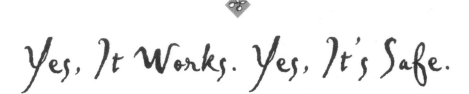

Yes, It Works. Yes, It's Safe.

Often when I am on talk shows the hosts pit me against nutritionists and doctors who believe in low-fat diets. It makes for good ratings if everyone is arguing, but it's hard to hear the truth through all that noise. Let me answer some important questions raised by the critics about the health benefits of Somersizing. Ahhh, no one can interrupt me in my own book.

Question #1: Shouldn't we be following the USDA Food Pyramid as the optimum guide for eating healthy?

The USDA recommends that on a daily basis we eat 6–11 servings of carbohydrates, 2–4 servings of fruit, 3–5 serving of vegetables, 2–3 servings of dairy, 2–3 servings of protein, and fats and sweets only sparingly. That breaks down into 60 percent carbohydrate, with 15 percent protein, and no more than 25 percent fat. Following this food plan will only make your body appear the same shape as the pyramid! As I've discussed, all those carbohydrates are responsible for sending our insulin levels through the roof, which packs on the pounds. Carbohydrates are used by our bodies only as a fuel source, and since our body can also use our fat reserves or the proteins we eat as a fuel source, carbohydrates are not considered an essential part of our meal plans. Fat and protein, on the other hand, create virtually no rise in insulin levels, and provide our bodies with the building materials needed for good health. Therefore, Somersizing recommends you turn the pyramid upside-down, eating mostly protein, fats, and vegetables, with minimal amounts of complex carbohydrates in the right combination with other foods. And when you do . . . watch your figure change shape, just like the turned-over pyramid!

Question #2: Isn't a low-fat diet the safest and most effective way to lose weight?

Noooooooooooooooooooooooooooooooooo ooooooooooooooooooooooooooooooooooooo oooooooooooo!

Let me explain why a low-fat diet can be dangerous to your health. As we've learned, we must eat protein and fat to make hormones that regulate the systems of the body and promote healthy cells. Proteins and fat are necessary for the constant rebuilding that takes place in our bodies. When we do not supply our body with these essential nutrients, our body will break down our *muscles* and *bones* to derive the materials it needs for rebuilding.

Although the scale may say you are losing weight on a low-fat, high-carbohydrate diet, you are actually losing more muscle and bone mass than you are fat! But, again, your body will kick into survival mode and slow down your metabolic processes to halt the depletion of your bones and muscle mass. It is at this point that you experience the tired feelings that accompany low-fat, high-carbohydrate diets. If you ever feel fatigue when dieting, be alerted that your body is not getting the food it needs to thrive! Low-fat diets deprive our bodies of the essential elements we need for living. If you lose weight, you are most likely losing muscle and bone mass. Again, when you go off the diet and resume your normal eating habits, you will gain back more fat than before.

Plus, muscle mass is necessary for helping to decrease insulin levels. Muscle provides another area for insulin to stow away ele-

vated blood sugar, so that it does not get converted to fat. By limiting proteins and fats in our diet, we decrease our lean muscle mass, which means that insulin has fewer places to store sugar. This leads to insulin resistance, which we know is the reason we pack on the extra pounds. Eating a low-fat, high-carbohydrate diet may initially decrease your body fat, but it will also decrease your lean muscle mass. Carbohydrates do not build muscle. Protein and fat, on the other hand, are *essential* to build muscle. If your diet is deficient in protein and fat, your muscle mass will become depleted. Less muscle mass leaves fewer places for sugar to be stored, so the carbohydrates you continue eating will be converted to fat and stored in the fat cells.

Question #3: How can we unload the stored sugar in our cells?

Somersizing encourages eating appropriate proteins, fats, vegetables low in starch, and fruit in proper combinations to unload the built-up sugar in our system. This unloading is the burning of fat stores. This is what I refer to as "The Melt." As our system unloads, we melt away our fat reserves until we find our ideal body weight. We lower our insulin resistance and begin to reprogram our metabolism. In addition, because you are giving your body essential nutrients, you are decreasing excess body fat while you build lean muscle mass. And by regulating the hormonal systems of the body, you will discover the key to preventing disease. How wonderful that eating delicious, flavorful, nutritious foods will help keep our

Dear Suzanne,

I just wanted to thank you for both of your books on Somersizing. I have lost about 25 pounds painlessly and am skinny again! I have people stopping me every day and asking me how I did it. I give your books all the credit and tell people how easy it is. While I have stuck to the food combining principles rigidly, I have skipped between Level One and Level Two frequently and still had no trouble losing weight.

I also feel better than I ever have! I am sleeping better, getting up earlier, sometimes before my alarm rings (this has never happened in my life!) and have much more energy. I was aware I had a sensitivity to wheat so I knew I felt better when I stayed away from that. I found I felt better when I stayed away from carbohydrates in general and just ate meat, chicken, fish, some dairy and veggies and fruits (and red wine and chocolate!).

So, thank you. I found the books very easy to follow, but I have been interested in and exploring these issues for years.

Thanks again and all the best,
Wendy Twomey

P.S. It has now been five months since I wrote you and eight months since I lost the weight and I've had no problem keeping it off. In fact, I'm enjoying the "fattening" foods I haven't indulged in for years. I love it!

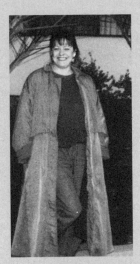
before

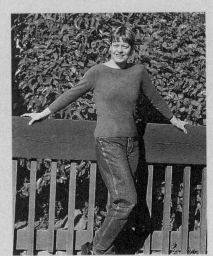
after

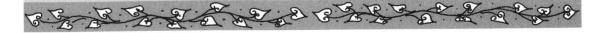

insulin levels stabilized, so we can lose weight and slow down the aging process.

Some people will experience The Melt faster than others. Some people see amazing results in the first week. Hundreds of people have told me they lost 25 pounds in the first month. For me it was not so fast. I Somersized for almost two months before I saw results, then one morning I woke up and The Melt had begun. The fat literally began melting off my body and I have never looked back.

Question #4: Can you overeat protein and fat?

Many people are concerned about eating too much protein and fat. I understand. It takes time to undo the brainwashing we have undergone in the past twenty years. Think about the diet of Eskimos. The Eskimo diet is made up of almost no carbohydrates. They eat mainly protein and lots of fat, yet they have almost no incidence of heart disease, high blood pressure, diabetes, or obesity. There was a study done in 1929 and 1930 following the diet of two Arctic explorers who ate nothing but caribou meat all winter long. They ate over 2,500 calories a day, with 75 percent of those calories coming from fat. Yet at the end of the year they had lost about 6 pounds, their cholesterol was normal, and they showed no ill effect from eating all protein and fat. It is the introduction of refined carbohydrates into civilized society that has caused the problems. You just cannot overeat proteins and fats. These foods are essential to life, and provide our bodies with the building blocks for good health.

The other wonderful news about protein and fat is that when you eat fat, your body releases a hormone called cholecystokinin (CCK) from the stomach. That hormone tells your brain you are satisfied and to stop eating. That is why people feel so satisfied after a Somersize meal. You are giving your body the food it craves and satisfying the hunger. If your metabolism could talk it would say, "Hey, thanks for the protein and fat. Now I have what I need to keep on truckin'. You can put the rest in the fridge." Carbohydrates, on the other hand, can cause you to eat and eat without ever feeling satisfied. So go ahead and eat hard-boiled or deviled eggs, or tuna salad with real mayonnaise, or little pieces of sausage and cheese. Not only will your body thank you for the essential proteins and fats, but you won't have that empty hungry feeling anymore!

Question #5: I'm worried about eating foods so high in cholesterol. Doesn't this put me at risk for heart attacks?

Increased cholesterol and heart disease is a huge concern for everyone. Talk to your doctor about the connection between raised insulin levels and heart disease. There are thirty years of medical studies to prove a correlation between the two. (See the next chapter for more information.) If your doctor is ignoring the effects of insulin, you must be proactive and find the information yourself. I hear the same story over and over again.

If you have high cholesterol, you've probably been hounded by your doctors and your family members to cut back on foods high in fat and cholesterol. But is your low-fat diet helping to lower your cholesterol? It's doubtful. Only 20 percent of the cholesterol found in your blood is a direct result of the foods you eat. The remaining amount is produced by your liver from excess sugars (carbohydrates). Although it seems logical that cutting back on fatty foods will decrease your total cholesterol levels, in actuality, the less fat you eat, the higher the rate of cholesterol production in the liver!

Cholesterol and fat are absolutely essential to good health. They are used by the body as building materials and are in need of constant replenishment from the foods we eat. Cholesterol is used to make important hormones such as estrogen, testosterone, progesterone, DHEA, and the antistress hormone cortisol. When we deprive our bodies of cholesterol, the compound the body uses to make these hormones, cell membrane structure is altered and cell growth is disrupted. This causes an increased risk of cancer because cancer arises from the abnormal division of cells. In addition, a lack of cholesterol in our diets can lead to depression and irritability.

Spread the word . . . we must include cholesterol in our diets to stay healthy! If we do not eat cholesterol, our body will produce its own cholesterol by converting the carbohydrates we eat into cholesterol. Again, insulin plays an important role in the cholesterol equation. Insulin activates an enzyme in your liver called HMG-CoA reductase, which causes your liver to overproduce cholesterol from the carbohydrates you eat. When insulin levels are high, the liver produces more cholesterol. It is this internal overproduction of cholesterol that contributes to the formation of damaging artery plaque that can lead to diseases such as heart attacks and stroke.

This dangerous pattern put my own husband at risk. As I shared with you in *Get Skinny,* Alan thought he was the picture of health, but when he went to the doctor, he was told his cholesterol level was dangerously high—255. His doctors, as one would expect, told him to cut back on foods high in cholesterol and fat. He explained that his diet was already low in fat and that he ate mostly fruits and vegetables. They told him to cut back the fat and cholesterol even more. Fearing for his good health, Alan cut out virtually all eggs, meat, and cheese that he used to enjoy in moderation in his regular diet. He cut back on the butter and cream. Essentially, his diet consisted of a lot of fresh fruit, fresh vegetables, and plenty of pasta with low-fat sauces.

Before too long I started noticing that Alan was getting a little paunchy around the middle. I told him all that fruit must be making him fat. He laughed. "Fruit doesn't make you fat," he'd say. "And besides, I have to watch my cholesterol." Surprisingly, when Alan went back to the doctor to have his cholesterol level checked, it had actually gone up! How could that be? He was eating little or no cholesterol and fat, yet his cholesterol had actually increased. The doctors were baffled and decided to put him on pills to lower his cholesterol.

Now it makes such sense to me! Alan's insulin levels were through the roof from the excessive amount of fruit and carbohydrates he was consuming. Alan was a victim of elevated insulin levels, which were causing weight gain (because the sugar was being converted to fat) and increased cholesterol (because he wasn't eating the necessary cholesterol his body needed, the enzyme in his liver caused his liver to convert the carbohydrates he was eating into cholesterol). The key to lowering Alan's cholesterol levels was to eat less fruit and pasta and to eat more foods with cholesterol and fat. And it worked. He is now off the medication and eating a more balanced diet, including moderate amounts of fruit, protein, fat, and complex carbohydrates, in proper combinations to keep his blood sugar levels balanced. Without the high insulin levels surging through his bloodstream, I'm happy to report that once again he's thin around the middle and his cholesterol levels are down within normal range.

When you Somersize, you are encouraged to eat real foods that help increase your HDL, the good cholesterol in your bloodstream. This good cholesterol is responsible for fighting off heart disease. Eating a diet too low in fat has been shown to lower your HDL. That's why when you Somersize, I encourage you to eat foods that increase your HDL—like olive oil, butter, and fish oil—and foods that help decrease your overall cholesterol—like lean meats, fresh fish, and unsaturated oils. Most important, you are controlling your insulin levels, which is the key to controlling cholesterol levels.

So those are the facts on fat and cholesterol. Make sure to include it in your meals by eating proteins/fats with vegetables and you will not gain weight or increase your cholesterol. In fact, you will lose weight because you will increase your metabolism and need more energy so you will be able to use your fat reserves. Plus, you will lower your cholesterol by eating the essential cholesterol and fat your body needs to thrive.

Question #6: I've never had a weight problem until now. Why am I suddenly struggling with my weight?

For many of us the way we once were able to eat when we were younger no longer works. Partly it is because of our sedentary lifestyles. Most of us drive to work, park in a subterranean garage, walk to the elevator, then walk from the elevator to our desks. That is pretty much the extent of our daily exercise. Our bodies are doing the best they can to metabolize the food we ingest (usually on the run), but there is no, or little, movement exerted to burn off the carbohydrates (which give us our energy) as fuel. When carbohydrates are not used as energy they are stored as fat. This is the reason I suggest eating carbohydrates (whole grain) in the morning, because it is more likely you will be exerting yourself somewhat during the day and burning the sugars as fuel. If you eat carbohydrates for dinner, it is unlikely you will exert yourself any further than walking to your favorite chair in front of the television set.

The second reason we gain weight is a slow metabolism. Some of us are born with a slow metabolism (those were the heavyset kids in school). These children were not necessarily eating more than the skinny kids, it's just that their metabolisms were not working at optimum. Because of this they were probably craving energy, and found relief in comfort foods, which are most often sugars and carbohydrates. As they ingested carbohydrates their adrenaline levels became pumped up, which then lowered their serotonin levels, which made them feel sluggish and tired and craving more carbohydrates; thus the beginning of the lifelong merry-go-round.

The next reason for a lowered metabolism is middle age. We lose our ability to metabolize our food quickly as we age. When our metabolism slows down, we have difficulty burning off our food efficiently as fuel. Somersizing helps to reprogram our metabolism to work as efficiently as it did when we were younger. In the case of a metabolism that never worked efficiently from the beginning, Somersizing helps reprogram it to do so. That is the beauty of this regimen; it reprograms your metabolism by balancing your hormones, in particular the hormone insulin, which is the fat-storing hormone. Somersizing empties your cells of stored sugars, leading to balanced insulin levels (you will know this has happened when you stand naked in front of the mirror and you are no longer thick around the middle). For these reasons it is vital that you really learn what foods the body recognizes as sugar: white flour; white rice; high-starch vegetables such as potatoes, beets, carrots, corn, sweet potatoes, yellow squashes, yams; natural sugars like honey and molasses; raw sugars; and of course, the sugars used in cakes, cookies, pies, and candy bars. (You'll find the complete list in the Funky Foods section.) In

giving up the sugars your insulin levels will become balanced. With Somersizing, although you cannot have these beloved sugars, you *can* have *real* fats with any meal that is protein and/or vegetables. Just think about it; this means butter, cream, sour cream, full-fat cream cheese, cheese, and olive oil; this means you can have sauces on your chicken, meat, or fish. Sauces are delicious; butter, wine, and lemon sauces; wine reduction sauces; deglazed sauces made with pan drippings and butter; cream sauces, cream-based soup, and so on. Forget all the fat-scare articles you have been reading; we need fat in our diets for healthy cell reproduction.

Question #7: But haven't there been many medical studies that show eating fat makes you fat and raises your cholesterol?

The answer is no! There are *no* long-term studies regarding the negative effects of fat. In fact, Dr. Schwarzbein explained to me how the entire "fat scare" possibly resulted from one lone study in 1981. A five-year study followed approximately 1,200 men who were healthy, but considered high risk for coronary heart disease because they smoked and had high cholesterol levels. Half of the men were placed in the intervention group and instructed to stop smoking, eat less sugar, drink less alcohol, and reduce their cholesterol intake. The other half in the control group were to continue eating, drinking, and smoking as they always had.

The intervention group had checkups every six months and were encouraged to continue a healthier lifestyle, including

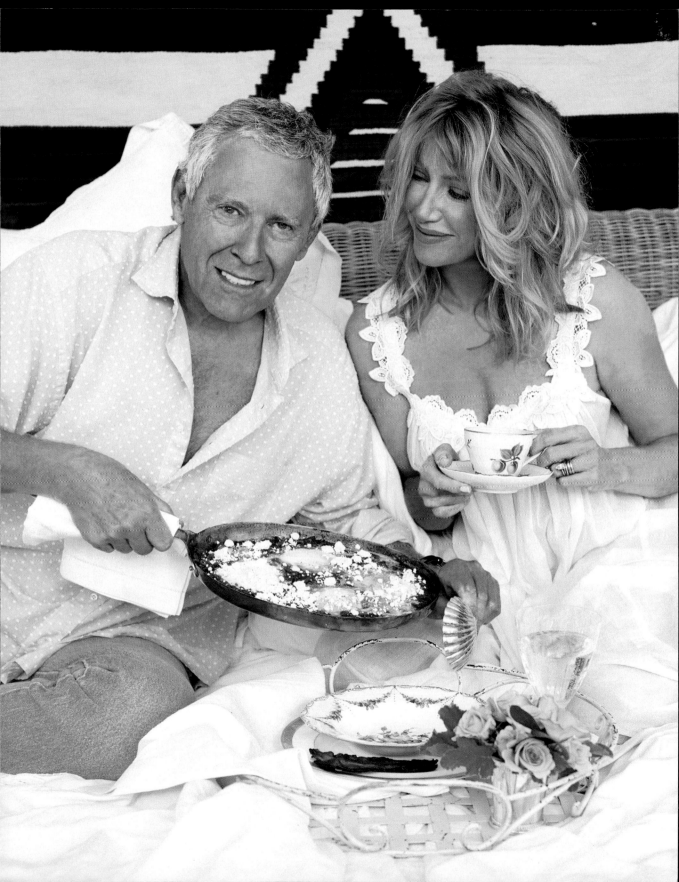

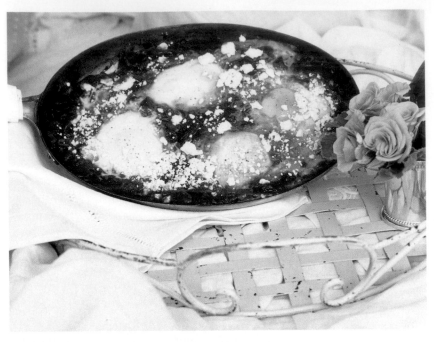

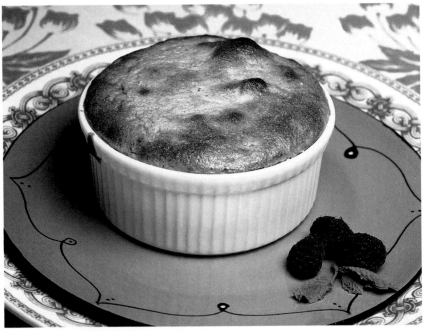

PREVIOUS PAGE AND TOP: Alan whips me up a scrumptious breakfast
in bed, with Eggs Baked in Tomatoes and Red Peppers.
BOTTOM: Raspberry Soufflé

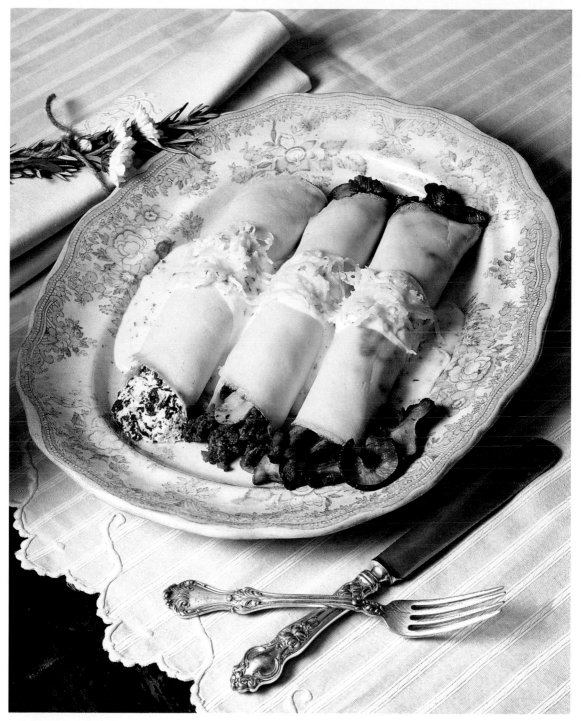

Egg Crêpes with Spinach and Ricotta Filling, Ground Beef Filling, Wild Mushroom Filling, and Creamy Parmesan Sauce

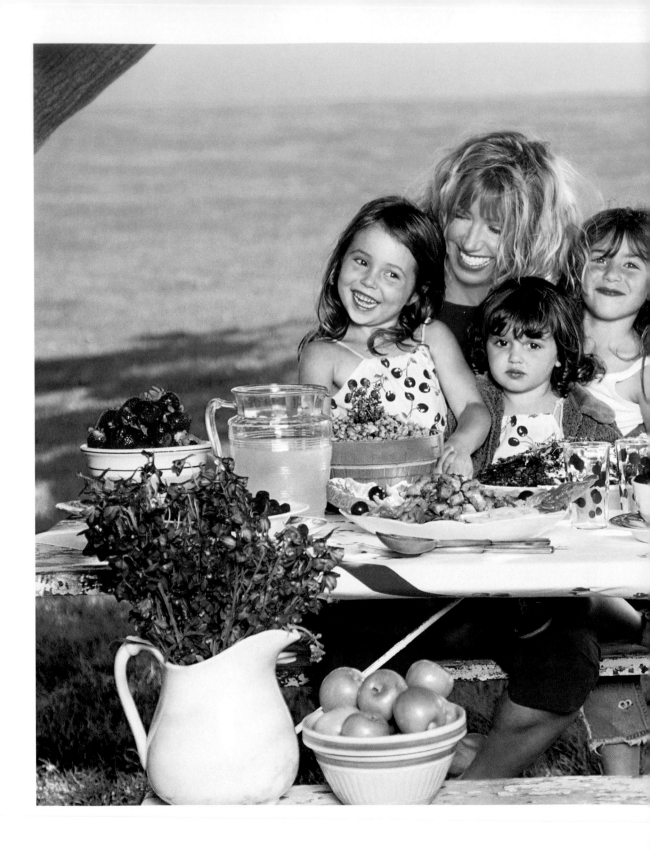

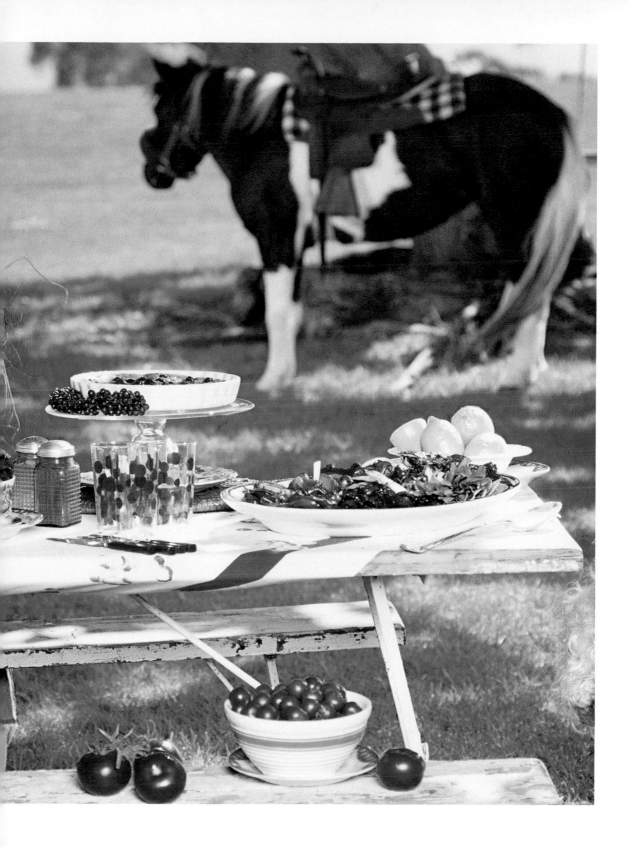

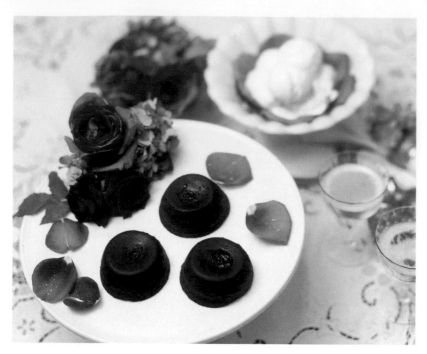

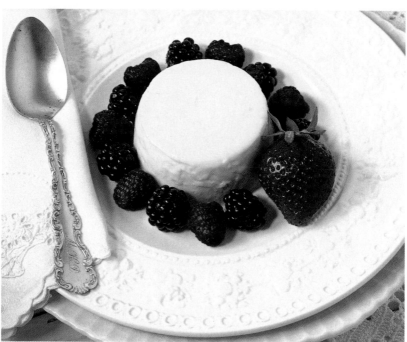

TOP: Molten Chocolate Cakes with fresh Vanilla Bean Ice Cream
BOTTOM: Panna Cotta with strawberries and raspberries
FOLLOWING PAGE: Southwest Christmas dinner with Deep-Fried Turkey and all the trim-
mings.

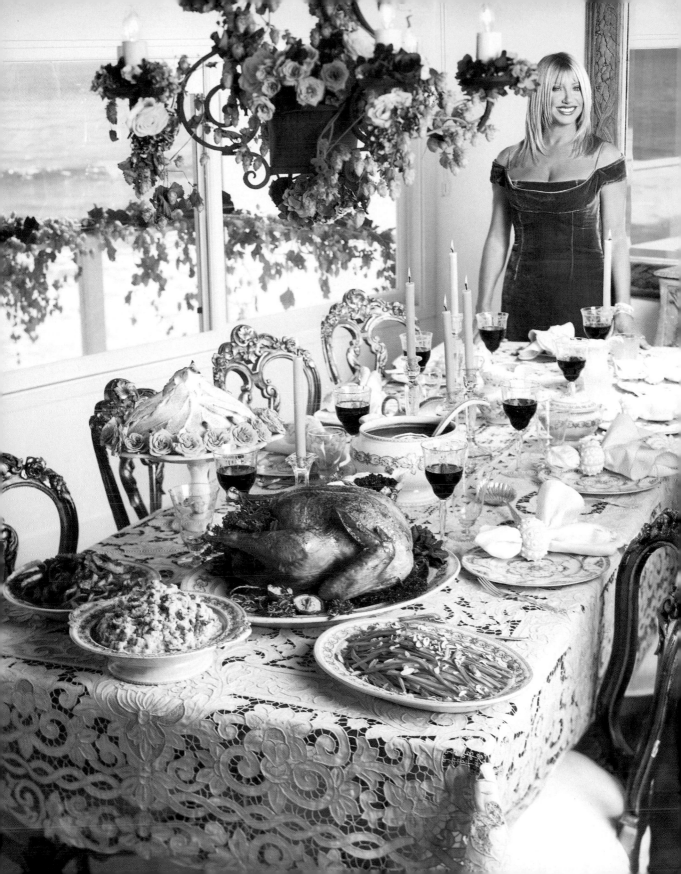

Zucchini Noodles

SERVES 4

These zucchini noodles are inspired . . . if I do say so myself! They are a great substitute for pasta and they are beautiful! You create long ribbons with your potato peeler. Chop up the leftovers to toss in soups or salads.

12 zucchini
2 tablespoons extra-virgin olive oil

Salt and freshly ground black pepper

With a good potato peeler, create long noodles by starting at the top of the zucchini and "peeling" wide ribbons down the length of the zucchini. Continue making ribbons as you turn the zucchini to get all the green part off first. When the center portion becomes too thin, set it aside and start a new zucchini. (Use the leftover centers in soups or salads.)

Heat a large skillet on medium high. Add the olive oil and the zucchini noodles. Sauté the noodles for 2–3 minutes. Season with salt and pepper.

Serving Suggestions

Zucchini noodles are a fabulous side dish for meat, fish, or poultry. Toss them with my Basil Pesto (p. 155). And make sure to try the wonderful recipe with Pan-Fried Garlic Lemon Shrimp (p. 214). Or you can have them with Meat Sauce (p. 238) and Meatballs (p. 239). Anywhere you'd eat pasta, you can substitute zucchini noodles.

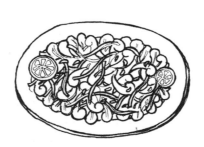

Black Bean Vegetable Chili

CARBOS AND VEGGIES—LEVEL ONE

SERVES 8

This chili is loaded with fresh vegetables and black beans. If you're using dried beans, they'll need to soak overnight. If you use fresh beans or canned beans, they need no preparation. This recipe contains no oil, so you can enjoy it on Level One as a great Carbos meal. For Level Two you can sauté the vegetables in olive oil and top the chili with cheese and sour cream.

2 cups black beans, dried or canned
1 eggplant, cut into ½-inch cubes
1 tablespoon coarse (kosher) salt
½ cup tomato juice (for Level Two: ½ cup
   olive oil)
2 onions, cut into ¼-inch dice
2 zucchini, cut into ¼-inch dice
1 red bell pepper, cored, seeded, and cut
   into ¼-inch dice
1 yellow bell pepper, cored, seeded, and
   cut into ¼-inch dice
1 large clove garlic, coarsely chopped
8 ripe plum tomatoes, cut into 1-inch
   cubes

1 cup vegetable broth
1 cup chopped fresh Italian parsley
½ cup slivered fresh basil leaves
3 tablespoons best-quality chili powder
1½ tablespoons ground cumin
1 tablespoon dried oregano
1 teaspoon dried red pepper flakes
½ cup chopped fresh dill
¼ cup freshly squeezed lemon juice
Salt to taste
Nonfat sour cream for garnish
3 scallions, white part and 3 inches green,
   thinly sliced, for garnish

To prepare dried black beans, rinse with water and pick out any debris. Place in a large bowl with enough water to cover by 2 inches. Soak overnight or for 8 hours. Drain the beans and place in a stockpot with fresh water to cover. Bring to a boil, then reduce heat and simmer for about 30 minutes, until tender. Strain the beans and set aside.

Place the eggplant in a colander. Toss it with the coarse salt, and let it sit for 1 hour to remove the moisture. Pat dry with paper towels.

Heat ¼ cup of the tomato juice (for Level Two, use olive oil) in a large flame-proof casserole. Add the onions, zucchini, bell peppers, and garlic. Sauté over medium low heat for about 10 minutes.

Place the remaining ¼ cup of tomato juice in a skillet, and cook the eggplant over medium high heat until just tender, about 10 minutes. Using a slotted spoon, transfer the eggplant to the casserole.

Add the tomatoes, broth, ½ cup of the parsley, basil, chili powder, cumin, oregano, and red pepper flakes to the casserole. Cook over low heat for 30 minutes, stirring occasionally.

Add the cooked beans, dill, and lemon juice. Cook another 15 minutes. Add salt to taste, adjust the seasonings, and stir in the remaining ½ cup parsley. Serve hot, garnished with a dollop of nonfat sour cream and scallions.

For Level Two
Use full-fat sour cream, grated cheese, and scallions

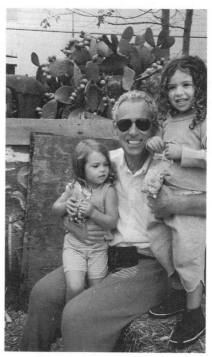

Alan with his girls.

Middle Eastern Vegetable Stew

CARBOS AND VEGGIES—LEVEL ONE

SERVES 6

This vegetable stew gets dressed up with curry powder and is then served over tabbouleh or brown rice. To enhance the flavor of your curry powder, or any bottled spices, sprinkle the powder in a dry nonstick frying pan and toss over medium heat for 2–3 minutes. You don't want the curry to color or burn, but you'll notice the increased fragrance. By heating the curry powder you release the natural oils.

4 cups vegetable stock
1 large onion, chopped
5 cloves garlic, minced
3 tablespoons whole wheat flour
1 pound pattypan squash, diced
3 medium zucchini, cut into ½-inch rounds
3 medium yellow zucchini squash, diced

4 stalks celery, thinly sliced
2 teaspoons dried oregano
1 teaspoon curry powder
4 Roma tomatoes, chopped
2 scallions, chopped
Salt and freshly ground black pepper
1 recipe Tabbouleh (p. 185) or cooked whole-grain pasta or brown rice

In a sauté pan, heat ½ cup of vegetable stock. Add onion and garlic, and sauté until translucent.

In a large Dutch oven or stockpot, mix the remaining 3½ cups of stock and the whole wheat flour. Bring to a boil, stirring constantly. Add onion mixture to the pan and reduce to a simmer. Stir in the squash, celery, oregano, and curry powder, and cook for 15 minutes. Add tomatoes and scallions. Continue to simmer until vegetables are tender when pierced with a fork. Season with salt and pepper.

Serve with Tabbouleh, whole-grain pasta, or brown rice.

Eggplant Parmesan

SERVES 6 – 8

You're not going to believe you can eat this and lose weight! There are many versions of this popular dish. The trick is not letting the eggplant get mushy. In this recipe you quickly fry the eggplant to keep it nice and crisp.

1 recipe Sweet Tomato Sauce (p. 235)
2 firm medium eggplants (about 2 pounds)
2 quarts peanut oil
Salt and freshly ground black pepper

1 pound mozzarella cheese, thinly sliced
1 cup freshly grated Parmesan cheese
½ cup loosely packed, roughly chopped
    fresh basil leaves

Preheat the oven to 400 degrees.

Prepare the Sweet Tomato Sauce and set aside.

Cut the eggplants lengthwise into very thin slices.

Heat the oil in a large skillet or deep fryer to about 360 degrees. Fry 2–3 slices of eggplant at a time until golden brown, about 4 minutes. Drain the slices on paper towels. Season with salt and pepper.

Spoon several tablespoons of the tomato sauce into a rectangular casserole dish (9 inches × 13 inches). Layer half the fried eggplant over the sauce. Spoon another thin layer of sauce over the eggplant. Cover with half the mozzarella, then about half of the Parmesan cheese. Layer the rest of the eggplant, then a little more tomato sauce, remaining mozzarella, and the other half of the Parmesan cheese. Sprinkle with the fresh basil.

Bake until the cheese is bubbling and melted, about 40 minutes. Let the casserole cool for about 10 minutes, then cut into squares and serve.

Fish and Seafood

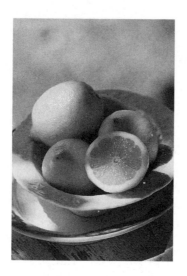

Clam Bake! Mussel Bake! Crab Bake! Lobster Bake!

PRO/FATS AND VEGGIES—LEVEL ONE

When I throw a party, I love to steam fresh clams, mussels, crabs, and lobsters in big pots right on the beach below my house. I serve the steamed seafood with loads of melted butter and fresh lemon.

Here's what you'll need:

Water
Clams
Mussels
Lobsters
Crabs
Cider vinegar
Old Bay Crab Boil

Melted butter
Lemon wedges

EQUIPMENT

Big stockpot with cover
Steam basket insert (that fits inside
   the big pot)

To cook clams and mussels, first rinse them in cold water to remove sand and dirt. When these mollusks are fresh, they are still alive. The shells will close automatically when they feel the cold water. If any shells are cracked, broken, or remain open, discard them.

Fill the large pot with 2–3 inches of water and layer the clams or mussels in the steam basket insert. Cover. Bring the water to a boil on high heat and occasionally shake the pan. It takes between 5 and 10 minutes to completely steam the mussels or clams. Peek in the pot and remove clams or mussels from heat when their shells are wide open. That means they are cooked.

To steam live lobsters, use the same method as above, but know that lobsters will take longer, about 15 minutes for a 1½-pound lobster. Fresh lobsters will change color from their natural speckled brown tones to a bright red. Increase the cooking time 2–3 minutes for every additional ¼ pound.

Many crabs today are precooked and then frozen. To refresh frozen crabs, place them in a pot of boiling water for 1–2 minutes and drain.

To steam live crabs you will also need a large pot with a steam insert. Add equal parts water to cider vinegar and fill the pot just slightly above the bottom of the insert. Layer the crabs with a sprinkling of Old Bay Crab Boil. Cover pot. Bring water and

vinegar to a boil and steam crabs until they turn bright pink and their legs can be easily pulled from their sockets.

Additional Suggestions

Create additional flavor when steaming your seafood by adding lemon juice or lemon slices, garlic cloves, dried herbs, or sprigs of fresh herbs such as parsley and thyme. Add bay leaves or black peppercorns. I often add dry white wine, a bottle of clam juice, or several tablespoons of white wine vinegar to the poaching water.

Red Hot Singing Scallops

PRO / FATS AND VEGGIES — LEVEL ONE

MAKES 18 APPETIZERS

Singing scallops are the small bay scallops from Canada. They make yummy little appetizers with a little mayo and hot sauce.

18 scallops, in the shell
¼ cup mayonnaise
8–10 dashes hot sauce (I like Cholula brand)

1 tablespoon finely chopped fresh parsley

Heat the broiler.

Open the scallops and discard the top shell. Arrange in a single layer on a baking sheet. In a small bowl, combine the mayonnaise with the hot sauce to reach your desired level of spice. Place a small dollop on each scallop. Sprinkle with a tiny bit of parsley.

Broil for about 3 minutes, or until the scallops begin to bubble. Serve immediately.

Crispy Fried Catfish with Ginger Chips

PRO/FATS AND VEGGIES—LEVEL ONE

SERVES 4

My son, Bruce, became a serious Somersizer this year. His wife, Caroline, came up with a lot of new recipes to keep him "thin and happy." This fried catfish has an exotic flavor, but it's easy to make and will knock your socks off.

1 bottle peanut oil (about 24 ounces)
1 recipe Green Goddess Dressing (p. 149)
1 large piece fresh ginger
4 cloves garlic
2 bunches cilantro
2 bunches scallions

Salt
Ground white pepper
4 catfish fillets
Soy sauce
1 lime, quartered

Heat the oil in a large frying pan on medium high heat until it reaches about 350 degrees.

Prepare the Green Goddess Dressing and set aside.

Peel the ginger, then thinly slice the root on an angle. (You should have about 20 slices.) Peel the garlic cloves and thinly slice on an angle. Wash the cilantro and trim off the ends. Wash the scallions and trim off the ends. To feather the ends of the scallions, lay each one on the chopping block and slice lengthwise, starting from the light green part down through to the white end. Then turn the scallions and slice again, creating a feathered end.

Begin the frying process with the ginger.

Fry the ginger slices until golden brown, about 4 minutes. Drain on paper towels. Add the garlic and fry for about 2 minutes. Drain on paper towels. Add the cilantro and fry for 2–3 minutes. Drain on paper towels. Add the scallions and fry for 3–4 minutes. Drain on paper towels. Salt each item to taste.

Sprinkle a little salt and white pepper on the catfish fillets. Add the catfish to the oil and fry for about 2–3 minutes, then flip and fry another 2 minutes. Drain on paper towels.

To serve, place a catfish fillet on each plate with a pile of ginger chips, fried garlic, fried cilantro, and fried scallions. Serve with soy sauce, a slice of lime, and a dollop of Green Goddess Dressing.

Grilled Ginger Shrimp on Skewers

PRO/FATS AND VEGGIES—LEVEL ONE

SERVES 6

Shrimp are a real crowd pleaser and a wonderful treat. I love to serve these on warm summer nights when my family comes for dinner. Even the grandchildren like the intense flavor the shrimp get from marinating all day. You may use fresh shrimp or flash-frozen shrimp. On the West Coast we have a chain of markets called Trader Joe's, and they carry flash-frozen fish. Ask your local fish market or grocery store if they can provide these. Anyway, this recipe is easy and delicious. Leave time so you can marinate it for a few hours so the flavors meld. Prepare about 10 shrimp per person.

60 uncooked shrimp (fresh or flash-frozen),
    peeled and deveined
1 large piece fresh ginger, peeled and
    thinly sliced
2 bunches scallions, chopped into 5-inch
    pieces
20 cloves garlic, peeled and sliced
2 cups peanut oil

1/2 cup soy sauce
1 teaspoon hot chili oil
2 tablespoons sesame oil
Freshly ground black pepper

EQUIPMENT

Bamboo skewers (at least 12)

Place the shrimp in a large bowl with all the other ingredients and let marinate for at least 2 hours in a cool place.

Prepare the grill.

Shortly before grilling, place the shrimp on bamboo skewers (about 5 shrimp per skewer). Reserve the marinated scallions to be grilled alongside the shrimp.

Heat a small frying pan on medium heat. Spoon out all the garlic and ginger slices and a ladleful of the oil in which the shrimp has been marinating, and fry the garlic and ginger for 2–3 minutes, or until golden brown and crispy. Set aside.

Place skewers on the hot grill and cook quickly, about 2 minutes per side. On the same grill, place the oil-soaked scallions and grill until crispy, about 2 minutes. At the last minute, carefully spoon some marinade over the shrimp, but please be careful because it causes the fire to shoot up.

Serve 2 skewers per person with a spoonful of the fried ginger and garlic, and a couple of grilled scallions.

Note

The shrimp can also be pan-fried. Just coat the bottom of a hot frying pan with some of the marinade and sauté the shrimp 2–3 minutes on each side.

Pan-Fried Garlic Lemon Shrimp with Zucchini Pesto Noodles and Arugula

PRO/FATS AND VEGGIES—LEVEL ONE

SERVES 6

I think just about all food tastes good cooked or coated in olive oil, lemon, and garlic. These shrimp are delicious served over zucchini ribbons that have been tossed in fresh basil pesto. Yum! I buy the flash-frozen jumbo uncooked shrimp that have been cleaned, deveined, and shelled, with the tails left on. I actually like these better than fresh shrimp because they have been flash-frozen immediately after being pulled from the sea, whereas fresh shrimp hang around the boat for a day, then have to be driven or shipped to the fish markets, so they actually are not as fresh as the flash-frozen.

60 uncooked shrimp (fresh or flash-frozen), peeled and deveined

3 cups olive oil plus some to drizzle on arugula

14 cloves garlic, sliced very thin

Juice from 3 to 4 lemons

1 bunch Italian parsley, stems removed and coarsely chopped

Freshly ground pepper

1 recipe Zucchini Noodles (p. 203)

Salt

1/2 cup Basil Pesto (p. 155)

8 ounces arugula leaves (or spinach leaves)

Lemon wedges for garnish

Place the shrimp in a large bowl. Coat the shrimp with olive oil, garlic, lemon juice (reserve some to drizzle on the arugula), parsley, and pepper. Gently toss to distribute flavor. Marinate for at least 2 hours in a cool place. Stir occasionally to marinate evenly.

Prepare the Zucchini Noodles and toss them in Basil Pesto. Arrange the zucchini noodles on individual dinner plates. Arrange a few arugula leaves around the edge and drizzle with a little olive oil, lemon juice, salt, and pepper. Set these plates aside while you prepare the shrimp.

Heat a large frying pan, then ladle as many shrimp as will fit flat, along with a few tablespoons of the marinade, into the hot frying pan. Using a slotted spoon, gather up all the garlic and parsley and include it with the cooking shrimp. Cook the shrimp quickly, 2–3 minutes on each side, and then remove from heat.

Season shrimp with salt. Place the shrimp in the middle of the zucchini noodles with a spoonful of the golden brown garlic. Garnish with lemon wedges.

Orange Roughy with Mushroom Stuffing

PRO/FATS AND VEGGIES—LEVEL ONE

SERVES 4

This baked fish is stuffed with a delightful mushroom filling, then topped with a red wine butter sauce.

FOR THE FISH

1½ pounds orange roughy (about 12 thinly
  sliced fillets)
Salt and freshly ground black pepper

FOR THE STUFFING

4 tablespoons butter
¾ teaspoon dried oregano
1 pound assorted fresh mushrooms,

roughly chopped
5 cloves garlic, minced
4 ounces cream cheese, room temperature

Olive oil

1 recipe Red Wine Butter Sauce (p. 157)

EQUIPMENT

Wooden toothpicks

Preheat oven to 350 degrees.

Season fish fillets with salt and pepper and set aside. Melt the butter in a large sauté pan, and add oregano. Add mushrooms and cook for 5 minutes, stirring constantly. Add garlic and continue to cook until most of the moisture has evaporated, about 10 minutes. Remove from heat, salt and pepper to taste, and let cool for 15 minutes.

Place mushroom mixture and cream cheese in the bowl of a food processor. Pulse until mixture forms a coarse paste.

Lay out fish fillets, skinned side down, and spoon about 2 teaspoons of mushroom filling onto each. Spread evenly. Starting from the narrow end, roll up each fillet and secure it with a toothpick. Place rolled fillets standing on their side in a baking dish. Drizzle with olive oil. Cover pan with foil and bake for 12–15 minutes. Remember to remove the toothpicks before presenting the fish fillets.

Serve with Red Wine Butter Sauce.

Pan-Fried Petrale Sole with Lemon, Butter, and Caper Sauce

PRO/FATS AND VEGGIES—LEVEL ONE

SERVES 2

I was raised in San Francisco, where petrale sole was abundant and anticipated. In my first autobiography I mentioned petrale sole often as one of the dinners I was able to afford on a regular basis to feed my son, Bruce. At that time I was able to get two slices of fresh fish for the two of us for about 80 cents. Alas, the cost of living has gone up and fish is no longer an inexpensive meal to put out for your family; but it continues to be a light, easy-to-prepare, healthful, and delicious choice. This is how I prepared sole back then, and I still do to this day. When fish is fresh, it needs very little adornment. Petrale sole is indigenous to the West Coast of our country. Any variety of sole will work for this recipe.

4 pieces of petrale sole
Salt and freshly ground black pepper
3 tablespoons olive oil
Juice from 1 lemon

3 tablespoons butter
1 tablespoon capers (optional)
Lemon wedges for garnish

Season both sides of the fish with salt and pepper.

Heat a frying pan on medium high heat. Add the olive oil to cover the bottom of the pan. When oil is hot but not smoking, add the fish pieces. Cook 2–3 minutes on each side, until fish is brown and crispy. Turn the fish over with a spatula and cook another 2–3 minutes on the other side.

Pour lemon juice over the fish and remove from pan. Set aside. Add butter and capers to the hot pan. Swirl butter until melted, scraping any bits off the bottom of the pan. Spoon butter sauce and capers over the fish and serve immediately with lemon wedges.

Poultry

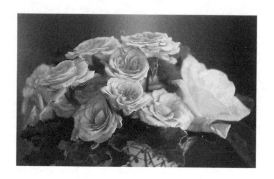

Pesto Fondue with Sausages

PRO/FATS AND VEGGIES—LEVEL ONE

SERVES 4

Warm, bubbling pesto with bite-size sausages dipped into it is absolutely delicious. This is a real crowd pleaser and a simple, easy addition to a fondue party.

1 recipe Basil Pesto (p. 155)
¼ cup olive oil

4–6 chicken sausages (or your favorite kind of sausage)

In a fondue pot, begin to heat the pesto and olive oil.

In a skillet, fry the sausages until cooked through. Let cool slightly, then cut them into bite-size pieces.

When pesto is cooked and bubbling, skewer the bite-size pieces of sausage and dip into the pesto.

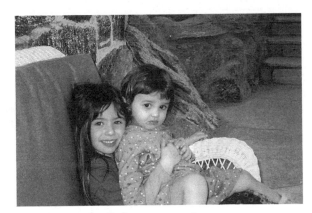

A big cousin hug.

Buffalo Wings with Blue Cheese Dip

MAKES 3 DOZEN PIECES

Would you believe little fried chicken wings with finger-lickin' spicy sauce and blue cheese dip are a Level One Somersize treat? For dinner I serve them with vegetable sticks and a big salad. For an appetizer I make plenty because they get gobbled up in seconds!

36 chicken drummettes (the small
   drummette from the wing)
2 tablespoons salt
2 tablespoons paprika
1 tablespoon cayenne pepper
3 cups peanut oil
⅓ cup hot sauce (the bright orange sauce made from red peppers, such as Cholula brand)
2 tablespoons butter
1 head celery, cut into 5-inch sticks
1 zucchini, cut into 5-inch sticks
1 head broccoli, lightly steamed
1 recipe Blue Cheese Dip (p. 146)

Place the drummettes in a bowl and toss with the salt, paprika, and cayenne.

Place the oil in a skillet; there should be about 2 inches in the bottom of the pan. Heat over medium heat until the oil reaches approximately 375 degrees. Fry about 8 wings at a time in the hot oil until crisp—about 10 minutes. (If you have a deep fryer, you can fry more wings at the same time.) Remove from oil and drain on paper towels.

Heat the hot sauce and butter over medium low heat until well combined.

Traditional buffalo wings are completely coated in the hot sauce, then served with blue cheese dip. I like to serve the wings with a bowl of hot sauce and a bowl of blue cheese dip on the side. That way the wings stay nice and crisp and you can control the amount of hot sauce on each bite. (Plus, your fingers don't get so messy).

Serve with the celery and zucchini sticks and broccoli florets.

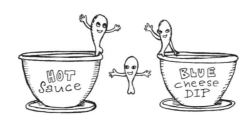

Deep-Fried Turkey with Fried Onions and Herbs

PRO/FATS AND VEGGIES—LEVEL ONE

SERVES 8–10

This is my favorite recipe of the year. I'd been wanting to try this Southern delicacy for so long. Recently I found a deep fryer for this purpose at Home Depot. It's a tall, narrow stockpot fitted with a stand or a basket to safely lower the bird into the hot oil. It also comes with a thermometer and spicy Cajun seasoning. With this method you can cook a 16-pound turkey in less than an hour! It comes out beautifully browned and crispy on the outside, moist and tender on the inside. You've never tasted turkey this great! Try it with my Roasted Turkey Gravy (p. 158). The initial investment of the pot and the peanut oil is worth the money. You won't believe what a winner this is.

9–10 quarts peanut oil
1 16-pound turkey
Prepared Cajun seasoning or poultry
   seasoning

Salt and freshly ground black pepper
8 onions, thinly sliced into rings
Bunches of fresh sage, parsley, Italian
   parsley, basil

Heat the oil in the stockpot until thermometer reads 350 degrees.

Rub the turkey liberally with the Cajun seasoning. Or season with salt, pepper, and poultry seasoning. Place the turkey on the provided stand or in the basket. When oil is hot, turn off the heat, then carefully lower the turkey into the hot oil. Turn the heat back on and cook 3 to 3½ minutes per pound (about 1 hour for 16 pounds). To remove the turkey, turn off the heat, then pull the bird out using the handle. Set aside.

Turn the heat back on. Add about half the onions to the hot oil and fry until golden, about 3 minutes. Drain on paper towels. Repeat with the other half of the onions. To fry the herbs, tie them in bunches using kitchen string, so that each bouquet has sage, basil, and both kinds of parsley. Drop the bouquets into the oil, 3 or 4 at a time, and cook for 3–4 minutes. Drain on paper towels.

Serve the sliced turkey with a pile of fried onions and an herb bouquet per person.

Lemony Chicken Burgers

PRO/FATS AND VEGGIES—LEVEL ONE

SERVES 6

These tangy little chicken burgers really hit the spot. Serve them with a big helping of vegetables and lots of lemon wedges.

1 pound ground chicken
1 large onion, finely chopped
4 cloves garlic, minced
1 egg, beaten
1 tablespoon grated lemon zest
2 tablespoons lemon juice
3 tablespoons chopped fresh parsley

2 tablespoons olive oil
1 teaspoon caraway seeds, crushed
1^3/$_4$ teaspoons salt
^{1}/$_2$ teaspoon freshly ground black pepper
Peanut oil for frying
12 lemon wedges for garnish

Mix all ingredients except peanut oil and lemon wedges in a bowl. Form the chicken mixture into 6 patties.

Heat peanut oil in a large skillet over medium heat. Fry the patties for 5–6 min-utes on each side, until crispy and golden brown.

Serve with fresh lemon wedges. Squeeze lemon on burger just before eating.

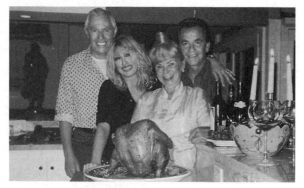

Yummy! I made Deep-Fried Turkey for Dick Clark's birthday.

Flattened Chicken

PRO/FATS AND VEGGIES

LEVEL ONE

This Tuscan-style chicken is crispy, easy, and delicious. You put a lid over the flattened chicken and then a large stone or a brick on top of that to flatten. The rest is easy.

1 4-pound free range chicken, butterflied
   (see below)
Salt and freshly ground black pepper
Paprika

2 tablespoons chopped fresh rosemary
   (or 1 tablespoon dried)
¾ cup extra-virgin olive oil
6 sprigs fresh rosemary

Have your butcher butterfly the chicken by slicing the backbone, then opening the chicken and flattening it.

Season both sides of the bird with salt, pepper, paprika, and rosemary. Heat the oil in an oversize skillet on medium high heat. When the oil is hot, place the chicken, skin side down, into the skillet. Put a lid over the chicken, then weight it with a heavy stone or brick.

Cook for about 15 minutes, until the skin is golden brown. Remove the weight and the lid. Turn over the bird and replace lid and weight. Cook for another 12 minutes. Chicken is done when the juices run clear.

Let it rest for about 10 minutes, then carve and serve. Garnish with rosemary sprigs.

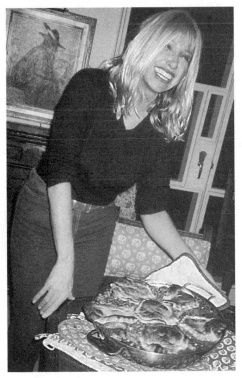

A little cheat with Chicken Pot Pie.

Chicken Breasts with Sage

PRO/FATS AND VEGGIES—LEVEL ONE

SERVES 4

I'm always looking for new ways to prepare chicken. This recipe is easy and delicious. It's best with fresh sage, but if you have a hard time finding it you may use dried. Consider growing a little herb garden in small pots. You'll love having access to fresh herbs.

4 boneless, skinless chicken breasts
Salt and freshly ground black pepper
Juice from 3 lemons
6 tablespoons extra-virgin olive oil

40 fresh sage leaves (or 2 teaspoons dried)
4 tablespoons unsalted butter
4 lemons wedges for garnish

Season the chicken breasts with salt and pepper. Place them in a casserole dish. Add the lemon juice, half of the oil, and the sage leaves (or dried sage). Turn the chicken to coat evenly, cover, and set aside at room temperature for 30 minutes.

Heat a large skillet on medium heat. Add the butter and the remaining 3 tablespoons of oil. When hot and bubbly, take each piece of chicken out of the marinade (reserving marinade and sage leaves) and place in the skillet. Cook until golden brown, about 5 minutes. Turn the chicken breasts over, then take the sage leaves out of the marinade and add them to the bottom of the skillet. Cook another 5–7 minutes until breasts are cooked through. The sage should get nice and crispy in the bottom of the pan. (If it is getting overcooked, remove it from the pan and set aside.) Remove the chicken breasts and sage leaves and cover loosely with foil while you make the sauce.

Return the pan to medium high heat. Add the reserved marinade and stir with a wooden spoon, scraping up the brown bits from the bottom of the pan. Let the sauce boil until it reduces to a thick syrupy sauce, about 1 minute. Pour the sauce over the chicken. Garnish with the lemon wedges. Serve immediately.

Chicken with Goat Cheese and Balsamic Syrup

PRO/FATS AND VEGGIES—LEVEL ONE

SERVES 4

This recipe was created when I thought I had nothing in the house to cook. Hmmmm . . . chicken, goat cheese, basil, balsamic vinegar, and Voilà! An amazing dinner!

2–3 tablespoons olive oil
10 cloves garlic, minced
11 ounces goat cheese
½ cup plus 1 tablespoon balsamic vinegar
14 fresh basil leaves, julienned, plus extra
    for garnish

Salt and freshly ground black pepper
4 boneless, skinless chicken breasts
1 tablespoon butter

Preheat oven to 400 degrees.

Heat a small sauté pan on medium low heat. Add 1 tablespoon olive oil and the minced garlic. Sauté garlic for about 1 minute until just golden. Remove from heat and place the garlic and remaining oil in a mixing bowl.

Add the goat cheese, 1 tablespoon balsamic vinegar, and the basil to the garlic. Mash together with a fork and set aside.

Heat a large sauté pan on medium high heat. Sprinkle the chicken breasts with salt and pepper. Add about 2 tablespoons olive oil, then the chicken to the pan. Cook for 4–5 minutes until golden brown on each side, then remove pan from heat. (Save the pan to make the sauce.) Remove the chicken breasts and place them in a casse-role dish. Generously spread the goat cheese mixture over each breast, dividing it equally among the four breasts. Place the casserole in the oven for about 5 minutes while you prepare the sauce.

Place the pan back on medium high heat. When hot, add ½ cup balsamic vinegar. Scrape the bits off the bottom of the pan to release the flavor. Reduce the sauce for about 1 minute until thick and syrupy. Turn off the heat and add the butter, stirring until well combined.

Remove the chicken breasts from the oven. The goat cheese should be a little melted so that it's soft. Drizzle the balsamic syrup over the breasts, garnish with a fresh basil leaf, and serve immediately.

Chicken Cacciatore

PRO/FATS AND VEGGIES—LEVEL ONE

SERVES 2–4

Cacciatore means "hunter" in Italian. You'll be glad you caught this one.

1 3½-pound whole chicken, cut up
Salt and freshly ground black pepper
¼ cup olive oil
1 medium onion, diced
1 bay leaf
1 teaspoon crushed dried rosemary
1 teaspoon dried oregano

8 ounces mushrooms, sliced
1 red bell pepper, seeded and cut into strips
2 cloves garlic, minced
½ cup dry red wine (see Note)
8 ounces tomato sauce
¾ cup Quick Chicken Stock (p. 161)
    or canned chicken stock

Season the chicken pieces with salt and pepper. Heat a large sauté pan on high. Add the oil, then the chicken pieces. Brown the chicken, about 5 minutes per side.

Remove chicken and set aside loosely covered with foil to keep warm. In the same pan, add onion, bay leaf, rosemary, and oregano. Cook until the onion is golden, about 7–10 minutes. Add the mushrooms and bell pepper and sauté for another 15 minutes until the vegetables are golden.

Add the garlic, wine, tomato sauce, and chicken stock. Bring to a boil, reduce heat to low, and place chicken parts back in pan. Cover the pan. Simmer 15 minutes, turn chicken pieces over, and continue to simmer for an additional 10–15 minutes. Add more salt and pepper to taste.

Note
Red wine creates a minor imbalance. If you are doing well on Level One, you should not have a problem.

Meat

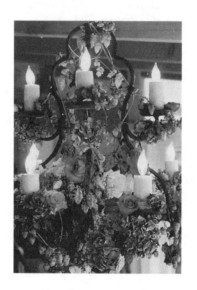

Pork Chops with Creamy Shallot Sauce

PRO/FATS AND VEGGIES—LEVEL ONE

SERVES 2

Whenever my grandaughters come over they always ask for these pork chops. They are sweet and yummy. Pork is one of those foods that really satisfies your hunger. I also love the flavor. Pan-fried pork chops leave you with wonderful bits on the bottom of the pan to make a sauce. This sauce is reduced with red wine and a little cream. In case you forgot . . . you're losing weight.

4 boneless center cut pork chops, 1 inch
   thick
Salt and freshly ground black pepper
4 tablespoons butter
1 medium onion, finely chopped

5 shallots, finely chopped
2 cloves garlic, chopped
1 cup red wine
1/2 cup heavy cream

Preheat oven to 200 degrees.

Season pork chops with salt and pepper. Heat a skillet on medium high. Melt 2 tablespoons of the butter in the pan. Cook chops for about 5 minutes, until the outside is golden brown. Turn them over and continue cooking for another 5 minutes. Remove pork chops from pan, and reserve in warm oven.

Add the onion to the skillet (and more butter if pan looks too dry) and cook until browned, about 7 minutes. Add the shallots and garlic and cook for an additional minute. Pour red wine into pan and bring to a boil. Turn the heat down to a simmer, and cook until wine has reduced by half, about 3–4 minutes. Add the remaining butter, stirring to melt. Whisk in the cream. Season with additional salt and pepper.

Return pork chops to pan, heat for 2 minutes in the sauce, and serve.

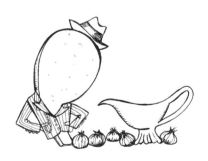

Rosemary Roast Loin of Pork

PRO/FATS AND VEGGIES—LEVEL ONE

SERVES 6

It is important to begin roasting this delicious roast pork at a high heat—to sear and brown the sur-face and help seal in the juices—then continue to roast gently at a lower heat, to cook it slowly with-out drying it out. Don't roast without the bones. They add essential flavor to the meat. But do ask your butcher to crack the bones, which makes it easy to slice the roast into thick chops at serving time. Serve this with Caramelized Fennel (p. 196) for an elegant meal.

1 loin end pork roast, bones split (about 5 pounds)
2 tablespoons olive oil
Salt and freshly ground black pepper
10 cloves garlic, minced

3 tablespoons fresh rosemary leaves (or 2 tablespoons dried)
About 1 1/2 cups dry white wine (see Note) (or 1 1/2 cups chicken broth)
About 1 1/2 cups water
3 tablespoons butter

Preheat the oven to 400 degrees.

Make several slits in the meatiest center section of the pork. Rub the roast with olive oil. Season it liberally with salt, pep-per, garlic, and rosemary. Place the pork, bone side down, on a roasting rack in a roasting pan. Place in the center of the oven and roast for about 30 minutes, until the skin is crackling and golden.

Reduce the heat to 325 degrees. Add 1/2 cup water and 1/2 cup wine and baste the roast by spooning the juices over the meat. If the juices dry up, add a little more wine and water as needed so that you always have some basting juices in the pan. Baste the roast about every 30 minutes. Roast the pork for 25 minutes per pound, or until a meat thermometer reads 155 degrees.

When finished, transfer the roast to a carv-ing block and cover with foil while you make the sauce.

Place the roasting pan on the stovetop over medium heat, scraping up all the brown bits to release the flavor. Add another cup of wine and 1/2 cup of water and reduce until the sauce is thick and syrupy, about 3–5 minutes. Turn off the heat and swirl in the butter.

Carve the roast into thick chops and serve immediately with the passed sauce.

Note

The white wine causes a slight imbalance, but if you are doing well on Level One, it should not be a problem for you.

Baby Back Pork Ribs

PRO/FATS AND VEGGIES—LEVEL ONE

SERVES 6

My family loves this dinner. I was never a big fan of ribs until I tried them this way. I've always found ribs too sugary; but for Somersize purposes, I think having them cooked as a savory is much more delicious. They are salty, and greasy in a good way. Everyone will be licking their fingers and asking for more.

6 racks baby pork ribs of 12 to 14 ribs each
    (to increase recipe, add more racks, but I
    find that one rack per person seems to
    satisfy)
Extra-virgin olive oil
Salt and freshly ground black pepper
1 bunch fresh thyme (or 2 tablespoons
    dried), chopped

1 bunch chopped fresh rosemary
    (or 2 tablespoons dried)
2 heads garlic, minced
Pinch of dried red pepper flakes
1 large lemon

Preheat oven to 375 degrees.

Fill a large stockpot with water and bring to a rolling boil. Add ribs and boil for 30 minutes.

Remove from water and place ribs side by side in a large roasting pan. Liberally rub ribs on both sides with olive oil and salt. Add pepper to both sides. Sprinkle top side with thyme and rosemary. Add minced garlic to cover ribs on top. Sprinkle more olive oil on top of crushed garlic (this makes the garlic crispy and wonderful). Season with hot red pepper flakes to suit your taste. (Remember, a little goes a long way.) Squeeze fresh lemon on top of this, and place roasting pan in hot oven. After about 15 minutes, carefully turn the ribs over to crisp up the bottom side and cook for an additional 15 minutes. Then turn over once again and scrape up any of the garlic and herbs that have fallen off, and spoon on top of ribs again. Cook for another 15 minutes. It should take a total of 45 minutes of cooking time. The ribs should look dark and crispy.

Serve each guest an entire rack cut into individual ribs.

MORE PLEASE!

Lamburgers

MAKES 4–6 BURGERS

These are yummy, spicy, and easy. Alan likes to makes them on our outdoor grill, but they taste just as great cooked in a frying pan. You can make them in the morning and let them rest in the refrigerator all day. This way the flavors have a chance to meld; but, again, this is not essential. They will also be delicious if they are freshly prepared.

1½ pounds ground lamb
1 teaspoon salt
1 onion, finely chopped
1 egg, beaten
2 teaspoons ground cumin
½ teaspoon ground allspice
½ teaspoon cayenne pepper
4 tablespoons coarsely chopped cilantro
   leaves

GARNISH

1 red onion, thinly sliced
Crème fraîche or sour cream
2 lemons, cut into wedges

Put the lamb, salt, onion, egg, cumin, allspice, cayenne, and cilantro into a food processor and process until well blended. Shape the mixture into 4–6 patties. Cook over a hot grill or in a frying pan for 5 minutes per side, or until they are well browned and cooked to your liking.

Serve with the red onion slices and a spoonful of crème fraîche or sour cream. Put a lemon wedge on each plate and serve immediately.

Lamb Loin with Tarragon Salsa

PRO/FATS AND VEGGIES—LEVEL ONE

SERVES 4

This incredible lamb dish was the entree at Jenny McCarthy's wedding . . . and I loved it. I think I have come very close to the caterer's guarded secret recipe. Maybe mine is even better!

½ cup diced tomatoes
7 tablespoons olive oil
2 tablespoons white wine vinegar
2 teaspoons chopped fresh tarragon

1 teaspoon salt
½ teaspoon freshly ground black pepper
2 pounds lamb loin for roasting

In a medium bowl combine tomatoes, 5 tablespoons of the olive oil, vinegar, tarragon, ½ teaspoon salt, and ⅛ teaspoon pepper. Set aside.

Preheat oven to 375 degrees.

Rub remaining oil, salt, and pepper on lamb loin.

Heat a skillet with ovenproof handle on high heat. Add a little more olive oil to cover bottom of the pan. Place lamb in the hot skillet and brown on all sides, about 5 minutes. Place the skillet in the oven and roast until meat thermometer reaches 130 degrees for medium rare, about 20–25 minutes. Remove from oven. Cover with foil and let sit 10 minutes. To serve, slice lamb on the diagonal and serve with a mound of salsa.

Grilled Marinated Lamb Chops with Lemon

PRO/FATS AND VEGGIES—LEVEL ONE

SERVES 4

My grandchildren love lamb chops. They nibble every tasty little bite off the bones. These chops are easy to prepare, even with a little tyke on your hip.

8 lamb chops, about ½-inch thick
¼ cup extra-virgin olive oil plus extra for the pan
3 tablespoons freshly squeezed lemon juice

Salt and freshly ground black pepper
Lemon wedges for garnish

Place the lamb chops, oil, and lemon juice in a plastic bag and marinate at room temperature for at least 30 minutes and up to 2 hours, turning from time to time. Remove the chops and set aside.

Heat a skillet over high heat or prepare the grill. Add a little olive oil to the pan. Add the lamb chops and cook for 2–3 minutes per side, until golden brown and a little crusty on the edges. Season both sides with salt and pepper. Serve immediately with lemon wedges.

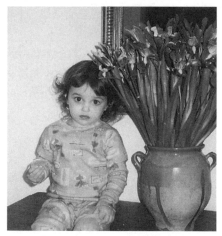

My youngest granddaughter eats three lamb chops!

Baby Lamb Chops with Parmesan Crusts and Sweet Tomato Sauce

SERVES 4

These thin little lamb chops are "breaded" with a tasty Parmesan crust and served with a sweet tomato sauce. These simple, flavorful meals are the essence of Somersizing.

Four eggs, lightly beaten
12 lamb chops, ½-inch thick
1 cup freshly grated Parmesan cheese
Salt and freshly ground black pepper

1 bunch fresh thyme (or 2 tablespoons dried)
3 tablespoons olive oil
1 recipe Sweet Tomato Sauce (p. 235)

Place the beaten eggs in a mixing bowl. Add the lamb chops and coat with egg.

Place the Parmesan in a shallow bowl. Dip each chop into the cheese, coating both sides.

Sprinkle both sides of chops with salt, pepper, and thyme.

It's best to place chops in the refrigerator for a couple of hours to allow the "breading" to set. (If you don't have time, you may omit this step.) Let the chops get back to room temperature before cooking (this will take about 1 hour).

Heat a large skillet, then add the olive oil to cover the bottom of pan.

Cook chops until Parmesan crusts are golden; then turn over to fry the other side, 2–3 minutes per side. The inside will be light pink and juicy.

To serve, spoon 2 or 3 tablespoons of Sweet Tomato Sauce in the center of each plate. Arrange 3 chops per person decoratively on top of sauce.

Serve immediately.

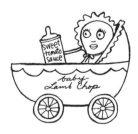

Sweet Tomato Sauce

PRO/FATS AND VEGGIES—LEVEL ONE

MAKES ABOUT 2 CUPS

This sauce celebrates the fresh clean taste of ripe tomatoes, garlic, and olive oil. It's pure pleasure.

1 large onion
8 fresh ripe tomatoes (or canned plum
  tomatoes, drained)

¼ cup good-quality extra-virgin olive
  oil
3 cloves garlic, minced

Chop onion in the food processor until finely minced. Coarsely chop the tomatoes in a food processor or blender.

Heat a medium skillet on medium heat. Add olive oil. When oil is hot, add minced onion and cook till translucent, about 4–5 minutes. Add the garlic and cook for another minute. Add the coarsely chopped tomatoes and reduce heat. Simmer for 45 minutes until sauce thickens a little.

Swiss Cheese Fondue

PRO/FATS AND VEGGIES—ALMOST LEVEL ONE

SERVES 4

Pull out your bell-bottoms; fondue parties are back! I've eliminated the cornstarch in this and added mayonnaise to bind the cheese and keep it smooth. I serve this with little bites of chicken, steak, broccoli, cauliflower, zucchini, and mushrooms. Add my Pesto Fondue with Sausages (p. 218) and Chocolate Fondue (p. 258) for dessert. Add some groovy music and your evening will be a sure hit.

FOR FONDUE

2 cups dry white wine (see Note)
8 ounces Swiss cheese, shredded
8 ounces Gruyère, shredded
1 cup mayonnaise
1/2 teaspoon dried mustard powder
1/4 teaspoon salt
1/4 teaspoon freshly ground black pepper
1/4 teaspoon nutmeg

FOR DIPPING

Bite-size pieces of cooked chicken breast
Bite-size pieces of cooked steak
Broccoli florets, blanched
Cauliflower florets, blanched
Zucchini chunks, blanched
Button mushrooms

In a large saucepan or heavy-bottomed pan, bring wine to a boil and reduce by half, about 10 minutes of simmering. Add cheeses, mayonnaise, and spices. Remove pan from heat, stirring constantly until all cheese is melted.

Transfer the cheese mixture to a fondue pot and set pan over an ignited alcohol or canned solid-fuel flame (if pan is ceramic, place a heat diffuser between it and heat source). Adjust heat so fondue bubbles very slowly. Check occasionally to be sure fondue is not scorching; if it is too hot, reduce or turn off the heat, then resume heating when mixture begins to cool.

Spear meat and vegetable cubes one at a time with fondue forks or thin skewers (metal or wood) and swirl through fondue (stir across bottom frequently to prevent scorching); lift out and let drip briefly over pan, then eat. If fondue gets too thick for easy dipping, stir in more heated wine, a few tablespoons at a time. After fondue is consumed, scrape the cheese crust from pan to divide and eat; it's considered a special treat.

Note

The 2 cups of wine in this recipe cause an imbalance. If you are doing well on Level One, you can probably handle this imbalance.

Meat Fondue

SERVES 4

This fun party food is making a comeback. In this fondue recipe you serve the meat raw, then dip it in the hot oil. Here's a recipe for beef, but you could certainly use chicken breast or lamb pieces, depending on your menu, guests' tastes, or the party theme.

Peanut oil for fondue pot

2 pounds steak, trimmed and cut into 1-inch cubes

Heat the peanut oil on the stove in a saucepan. Heat oil until instant-read thermometer registers 365 degrees. Carefully transfer oil from saucepan to fondue pot, and place in the holder. Using fondue forks, spear meat and cook in hot oil for 1–2 minutes, or until meat is done.

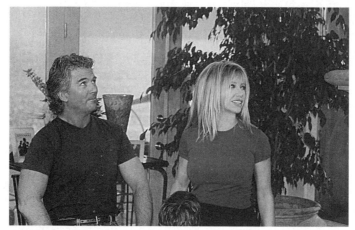

Patrick Duffy and I have remained close friends and often get together to eat great food and catch up.

Meat Sauce

PRO/FATS AND VEGGIES—LEVEL ONE

MAKES ABOUT 4 QUARTS

Every generation of Caroline's Italian family has cooked some form of this delicious meat sauce. Caroline learned from her mom, who learned from her mom, and so on. The ingredients were always measured in the palms of their hands . . . a pinch of this and a pinch of that. Caroline measured out all the spices, but feel free to add an extra pinch of this or that.

2–3 tablespoons olive oil
2 onions, chopped
1 head garlic, minced
2 pounds ground beef
1 tablespoon plus ½ teaspoon salt
2½ teaspoons freshly ground black pepper
2 teaspoons paprika
2 (28-ounce) cans tomato sauce
2 (28-ounce) cans tomato puree

1 (28-ounce) can peeled whole tomatoes, with their juice
2 tablespoons dried basil
2 bay leaves, cracked
½ teaspoon cayenne pepper
6 tablespoons finely chopped fresh parsley
½ teaspoon dried oregano
1 cup red wine

Heat a large stockpot on medium heat. Add the olive oil and onions. Sauté until the onions are translucent, about 7–10 minutes. Add the garlic and saute for 1–2 minutes longer. Add the ground beef and sauté until brown. Season the meat with about ½ teaspoon salt, ½ teaspoon pepper, and the paprika.

Add all 5 cans of tomatoes, roughly chopping the whole peeled tomatoes. Add 1 tablespoon salt, 2 teaspoons pepper, the basil, bay leaves, cayenne, parsley, oregano, and red wine. Stir all ingredients until well combined. Bring to a low boil, then lower heat and simmer for 1–4 hours. (The sauce will be ready after an hour but tastes better the longer you simmer it.)

For Level One serve over Meatballs (p. 239) and Zucchini Noodles (p. 203). For Level Two serve over whole-grain pasta with a sprinkle of Parmesan cheese. The meat with the whole-grain pasta creates an imbalance, but it's not as bad as it would be with white flour pasta.

Meatballs

MAKES ABOUT 24 MEATBALLS

Do you miss spaghetti with meatballs? This recipe comes from a long line of women in my daughter-in-law Caroline's family. Try these hearty meatballs with Meat Sauce and Zucchini Noodles. This combo will satisfy the biggest eaters.

Olive oil
1 pound ground beef
3 cloves garlic, minced
3 tablespoons finely chopped Italian parsley
2 eggs, lightly beaten

¼ cup freshly grated Parmesan cheese
3 dashes Worcestershire sauce (see Note)
Salt and freshly ground black pepper

Heat the broiler.

Drizzle olive oil on a baking sheet until the sheet is completely coated.

Combine the meat, garlic, parsley, eggs, cheese, Worcestershire sauce, salt, and pepper in a bowl. Use your hands to incorporate all the ingredients together. Form the meat into small round balls, about 1 inch in diameter. Place the meatballs on the oiled baking sheet. Broil for about 5 minutes, turning as necessary to cook all sides.

Serve on a bed of Zucchini Noodles (p. 203) covered with Meat Sauce (p. 238).

Note

Worcestershire sauce causes a minor imbalance. If you are doing well on Level One, you should not have a problem incorporating this small amount.

Jalapeño Chili

SERVES 8–10

This spicy chili is made with pork sausage, ground beef, and lots of jalapeños. I serve it with sour cream and Monterey jack cheese.

1 pound hot Italian sausages, cut into 1-inch lengths

1 pound sweet Italian sausages, cut into 1-inch lengths

¼ cup olive oil

2 cups coarsely chopped onions

6 cloves garlic, minced (3 tablespoons)

2 pounds ground beef chuck

2 green bell peppers, cored, seeded, and coarsely chopped

2 red bell peppers, cored, seeded, and coarsely chopped

6 jalapeño peppers (5 to 8 ounces total), cored, seeded, and cut into ⅛-inch dice; less if you don't want it to be too spicy

3 (35-ounce) cans Italian plum tomatoes, drained (5 cups tomatoes)

1 cup dry red wine (see Note)

1 cup chopped fresh parsley

2 tablespoons tomato paste

6 tablespoons best-quality chili powder

3 tablespoons ground cumin

2 tablespoons dried oregano

1 tablespoon dried basil

2 teaspoons salt

½ tablespoon fennel seeds

2 teaspoons freshly ground black pepper

2 pounds ripe plum tomatoes, quartered

Grated Monterey jack cheese for garnish (optional)

Sour cream for garnish (optional)

Sliced scallions, white part and 3 inches green, for garnish (optional)

Place a large, heavy skillet over medium heat, and sauté the sausages until well browned. (If necessary, add ¼ cup water while browning.) Transfer the sausages to paper towels to drain.

Heat a deep, heavy Dutch oven or stockpot with the oil over medium heat. Add onions and garlic, and cook until just wilted, 5 minutes.

Raise the heat to medium high, and crumble in the ground chuck. Cook, stirring frequently to break up the pieces, until the meat is well browned.

Add the drained sausages, bell peppers, and jalapeño peppers to the mixture. Cook, stirring frequently, until the peppers are slightly wilted, 10 minutes.

Stir in the drained tomatoes, wine, parsley, tomato paste, and all the herbs and spices (do not add the fresh tomatoes).

Cook for about 10 minutes, stirring frequently. Then add the fresh tomatoes and cook another 10 minutes.

Serve the chili in bowls, garnished with cheese, sour cream, and scallions if desired.

Note

Wine creates a minor imbalance. If you are doing well on Level One, you should be able to incorporate this small amount without a problem.

Hamburgers

PRO/FATS AND VEGGIES—LEVEL ONE

MAKES 6 BURGERS

Tasty meals don't have to be expensive or fancy. Select the hamburger with more fat content for the best flavor. Remember, when you Somersize, fat is your friend! These burgers are juiced up with garlic and herbs. Top them with your favorite cheese. I pile them with lettuce, tomato, dill pickle, mayonnaise, and a slice of red onion, then eat them with a knife and fork. If you're still hungry, have another! On Level Two you can also add a little ketchup.

2 pounds 80% lean ground beef
2 tablespoons chopped fresh parsley
4 cloves garlic, minced

1 tablespoon finely minced sweet onion
Salt and freshly ground black pepper
6 slices cheese (optional)

Preheat the grill to medium.

In a bowl, combine beef, parsley, garlic, onion, salt, and pepper. Mix until well blended. Divide into 6 portions (about ⅓ pound each). Hand-shape into patties about ¾-inch thick.

Grill burgers until browned on both sides, 2–3 minutes per side, and continue cooking until done to your liking. Top each patty with cheese, if desired, during last 2–3 minutes of grilling.

Beef Stew

SERVES 4–6

Beef stew is a wonderful winter comfort food. You won't find any potatoes or carrots in this version. I use celery, celery root, mushrooms, and onions in a tomato wine sauce. Light a fire and dig in.

1 tablespoon butter
4 ounces bacon
2 pounds trimmed beef round, cut into 1-inch cubes
1 onion, chopped
2 cloves garlic, chopped
3 stalks celery, chopped
1 medium celery root, chopped
12 pearl onions (see Note)

8 ounces whole button or other small mushrooms
1 bay leaf
1 teaspoon fresh thyme (or ½ teaspoon dried)
2 cups dry red wine
2 cups beef stock
1 cup tomato sauce
1 cup sliced green beans

Heat a large 6-quart Dutch oven or soup pot over medium high heat. Melt the butter, then add bacon and cook until pieces are brown. Drain on paper towels, then crumble and reserve.

Over high heat, sear the beef in the bacon drippings until light brown, about 3–4 minutes. Remove and reserve with bacon. In the same pan, add chopped onion and cook until translucent. Add garlic and cook for 1 minute. Add celery, celery root, pearl onions, and mushrooms, stirring constantly for about 5 minutes. Add the bay leaf, thyme, red wine, beef stock, and tomato sauce. Bring to a boil. Immediately turn heat down to a simmer, return bacon and beef to the pot, and cook covered for 20 minutes. Remove cover and add the green beans. Continue to cook until meat and vegetables are tender when pierced with a fork, approximately 15 minutes.

Note
For easy peeling, place the pearl onions in a bowl, cover with boiling water for 60 seconds, squeeze them, and the skin slips right off.

Beef Stir-Fry

PRO/FATS AND VEGGIES—LEVEL ONE

SERVES 4

This stir-fry will satisfy a hearty appetite with plenty of beef for the meat lover in your home. London broil is a nice cut of meat for this recipe, but your favorite steak will work just fine. The vegetables are stir-fried one at a time on high heat so as not to overcook them.

1¼ pounds London broil, sliced into
⅛-inch strips
3 cloves garlic, thinly sliced
1 cup peanut oil
Juice from 1 lemon
Freshly ground black pepper
3 cups chopped broccoli
3 baby bok choy, julienned

2 cups sliced mushrooms
1 cup julienned snap peas
2–3 tablespoons peanut oil
1 cup bean sprouts
¼ cup soy sauce
Dried chili oil for garnish
Hot red pepper flakes for garnish

Place the sliced beef, garlic, ½ cup of the peanut oil, lemon juice, and a few grindings of black pepper in a plastic zip-lock bag. Set aside and marinate for 20–30 minutes while you prepare the vegetables.

Heat a wok or large sauté pan over high heat. Add about 2 tablespoons peanut oil. Add the broccoli and sauté for 60–90 seconds. Place the broccoli in a large bowl and set aside. Then add the baby bok choy and saute for 60–90 seconds. Place the bok choy in the bowl with the broccoli. Add another tablespoon of peanut oil and the mushrooms. Sauté for about 2 minutes, then set aside with the other vegetables. Add the snap peas

to the pan (with a little more oil, if necessary) and sauté for 1 minute, then set aside with the other vegetables. Add the bean sprouts to the pan and sauté for 45 seconds, then set aside with the other vegetables.

Remove the marinated beef and garlic from the bag with most of the remaining oil and place in the hot pan. Sauté for about 2½ minutes until just cooked through. Add the vegetables back into the pan and toss everything together with the soy sauce for about 30 seconds. Place the stir-fry back into the bowl and serve immediately. For a spicy stir-fry, add a few drops of hot chili oil or a pinch of red pepper flakes.

Peppered Filet of Beef with Bourbon Sauce

PRO/FATS AND VEGGIES—LEVEL ONE

SERVES 4

This pepper steak has a wonderful sauce made from a reduction of red wine and a splash of bourbon. These are the little treats I allow myself on Level One. If you are steadily losing weight you should not have a problem with the minor imbalance caused by the alcohol. If you are just getting started and want to stay absolutely true to Level One, omit the alcohol and substitute a 14-ounce can of beef broth.

4 (5–6-ounce) filet steaks, trimmed
Salt
2 tablespoons black peppercorns, crushed
4 tablespoons butter

4 slices bacon
3 cloves garlic, chopped
²⁄₃ cup dry red wine
2 tablespoons bourbon

Season the steaks with salt. To crush the peppercorns, place them on a cutting board and crush them with the flat bottom of a skillet. Press your weight onto the skillet and smash the peppercorns. Sprinkle the steaks with the crushed peppercorns, pressing the pepper into the meat. Set aside.

Heat a medium skillet on high heat. Melt 1 tablespoon of the butter. Add the bacon and cook until crisp. Drain the bacon on paper towels. Cool, then crumble. Reserve.

Using the same skillet, turn the heat to high, and add steaks. For rare, cook 1½–2 minutes on each side. For medium rare, 2½–3 minutes on each side. Add more time for well done. Remove steaks to a platter and cover loosely with a piece of aluminum foil.

Add another tablespoon of butter to the skillet, over medium heat, and brown the chopped garlic for 1–2 minutes. Add the wine and bring to a boil. Stir constantly, loosening the brown bits on the bottom of the pan. Simmer the liquid until reduced by half. Turn off heat, whisk in the remaining 2 tablespoons of butter, and add the bourbon. Place the steaks on serving plates. Add the bacon pieces to the sauce, and drizzle the sauce over the meat.

Carne Asada de Perez

PRO/FATS AND VEGGIES—LEVEL ONE

SERVES 4

Oneida Perez is the extraordinary nanny for two of my granddaughters . . . and this is her extraordinary carne asada recipe from El Salvador, her home country. Serve it with her crunchy Salsa de Perez.

2 pounds skirt steak
2 bunches cilantro, roughly chopped
1 onion, roughly chopped
1 tomato, roughly chopped
1 cup freshly squeezed lemon juice

1 orange, sliced with peel (see Note)
Salt
1 recipe Salsa de Perez (p. 151)
Sour cream for garnish

Place the steak in a plastic bag or a nonmetallic bowl. Add the cilantro, onion, tomato, lemon juice, orange slices, and salt, making sure the meat is surrounded on all sides by the chopped vegetables. Place the bag in the refrigerator and let marinate overnight (at least 8 hours). Turn the meat once so that the lemon juice marinates both sides equally. Remove the meat from the marinade and discard the marinade.

Let the meat sit out at room temperature for about 30 minutes before cooking. Place the meat on a hot grill or under a broiler for 4–7 minutes per side. (Cooking time will vary depending on the thickness of the steak and how well-cooked you like your meat.)

Slice on the diagonal into thin strips. Serve immediately with Salsa de Perez and sour cream.

Note
The orange slices create a minor imbalance. You get most of the flavor from the tangy peel. If you are doing well on Level One, this minor addition should not create a problem.

Prime Rib Au Jus with Garlic Crust

PRO/FATS AND VEGGIES—LEVEL ONE

SERVES 4–6

What holiday would be complete without a perfectly prepared roast beef? There's no need to wait for a special occasion; I make this on Sunday nights and enjoy the meat throughout the week.

1 4-rib standing rib roast (about 7–8 pounds)
1 tablespoon olive oil
2 parsnips, chopped (see Note)
2 stalks celery, chopped
2 onions, quartered

FOR CRUST MIXTURE

3 tablespoons minced garlic
2 tablespoons Dijon mustard
1 teaspoon freshly ground black pepper

1 teaspoon salt
1 teaspoon crumbled dried thyme
1 teaspoon crumbled dried rosemary

FOR SAUCE

1 cup dry red wine (see Note)
2 cups beef broth

FOR GARNISH

Fresh rosemary sprigs

Preheat oven to 450 degrees. Let rib roast stand at room temperature for 1 hour before roasting.

In a large roasting pan, toss together the olive oil, parsnips, celery, and onions. Scatter the vegetables around the edges of the roasting pan.

In a small bowl, stir together crust ingredients until well combined. Set aside.

Place roast, rib side down, in the pan. Roast the beef for 25 minutes at high heat.

Remove roast from oven and turn the oven temperature down to 300 degrees. Using the back of a spoon, cover the "fat cap" with the crust mixture. Roast the beef slowly, for about 2–2½ hours, or until a meat thermometer registers 135 degrees for medium rare.

Transfer the roast to a cutting board and loosely cover to keep warm. (It's best to let the roast "rest" for 30 minutes before carving.)

While the roast is resting, make the sauce by placing the roasting pan with the vegetables on the stovetop over medium high heat. Remove the vegetables and discard. When the pan is hot, add the wine and broth. Scrape the bits off the bottom of the pan

with a wooden spoon. Let the sauce reduce by half, until it gets thick and syrupy.

Carve the meat and arrange on a platter. Garnish with rosemary sprigs. Serve with the delicious sauce on the side.

Note

Parsnips and wine create a minor imbalance. If you are doing well on Level One, you should not have a problem.

Florentine Steak

PRO/FATS AND VEGGIES—LEVEL ONE

SERVES 4

Alan used to have high cholesterol. He gave up all red meat, thinking it was creating the problem, but it only got worse. I finally convinced him to Somersize . . . he lost 20 pounds and lowered his cholesterol eating all the foods he thought he had to avoid. This steak is one of his favorites. I love to feed my husband. And I love knowing he's staying healthy with every delicious bite.

¼ cup extra-virgin olive oil
12 cloves garlic, thinly sliced
4 sprigs fresh rosemary
4 sprigs fresh oregano

4 sprigs fresh thyme
1 40-ounce porterhouse steak, at room
    temperature
Salt and freshly ground black pepper

Preheat the broiler.

Heat a skillet over medium heat. Add the olive oil and heat until hot but not smoking. Add the garlic, rosemary, oregano, and thyme. Cook until garlic is golden, about 1–2 minutes. Set aside to cool.

Season the steak liberally with salt and pepper. Place on a broiling pan and set under the broiler for 3–4 minutes per side (or until done to your liking). Transfer to a large plate.

Pour garlic, herbs, and oil over steak. Let steak rest about 10 minutes. Slice on the diagonal and serve each plate with some of the garlic and herbs.

Desserts

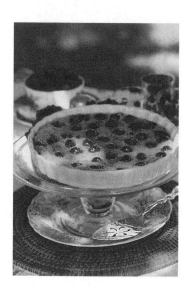

Vanilla Bean Ice Cream

MAKES ABOUT 1 PINT

It's ice cream! It's Level One!! It's made without sugar and without chemical sweeteners!!!! Do you love me, or what? It's a good time to invest in an ice cream maker. I use real vanilla beans for awesome flavor, and I love the little black specks in the ice cream. If you can't find vanilla beans, or don't want to spend the money, you can substitute vanilla extract.

2½ cups heavy cream
½ cup water
2 whole vanilla beans, scraped (or 1
    tablespoon vanilla extract)

4 teaspoons SomerSweet (or 2 teaspoons
    saccharin)
8 egg yolks

Pour ½ cup cream and the water into a saucepan. To scrape the vanilla beans, use the tip of a sharp knife to split the vanilla bean lengthwise. Scrape at the little black seeds with the tip of your knife. Drop them into the cream. Add SomerSweet, egg yolks, and vanilla bean hulls. Over double boiler, stir until everything is mixed together and heated through thoroughly. Do not boil. Add remaining 2 cups of cream and stir until heated thoroughly. Remove vanilla bean hulls. Pour into a bowl and place a piece of waxed paper over the top (right on top of the custard). Chill for 2 hours, then pour into ice cream maker and follow manufacturer's directions.

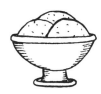

Dark Chocolate Ice Cream

PRO/FATS—ALMOST LEVEL ONE

MAKES 3 PINTS

This amazing ice cream is made from cream and eggs. It's so rich and thick, you only need a small bowl. The unsweetened chocolate creates a minor imbalance, but if you are doing well on Level One, you should not have a problem enjoying a bit of this after a Pro/Fats meal. You'll need an ice cream maker, but I'm sure you won't mind making the investment.

7 ounces unsweetened chocolate, chopped
5 egg yolks
3 teaspoons vanilla extract
5 cups heavy cream

2 tablespoon plus 2 teaspoons SomerSweet
(or 1 tablespoon plus 1 teaspoon
saccharin)

Place chocolate in a mixing bowl and reserve.

Whisk egg yolks and vanilla in another mixing bowl until pale yellow, about 3–4 minutes.

Warm cream in a medium saucepan over medium heat to 110 degrees or until bubbles form along the edge, just before boiling. Slowly pour hot cream into egg yolks, stirring constantly. Return to the saucepan and stir over medium heat until the custard thickens or it coats the back of a spoon. Add the SomerSweet and stir until well combined. Pour the hot mixture over the chopped chocolate, stirring until smooth.

Allow the chocolate custard to cool to room temperature. Refrigerate it, loosely covered, a minimum of 3 hours. Transfer to an ice cream maker, and freeze according to manufacturer's directions.

Sugarless Fudgysicle

MAKES 10

It's creamy chocolaty ice cream on a stick; and it's made with SomerSweet, so it's practically free! Only the chocolate creates a small imbalance. If you're doing well on Level One, you should be able to enjoy this treat every now and then without having a problem. You'll need 10 Dixie cups and Popsicle or wooden craft sticks if you don't have plastic molds.

1 ounce unsweetened chocolate
3 teaspoons SomerSweet (or 2 teaspoons saccharin)

2 cups heavy cream, well chilled
3 tablespoons unsweetened cocoa powder
2 teaspoons pure vanilla extract

Line 10 Dixie cups with plastic wrap so that the entire cup is covered, with a couple inches hanging over the edges. (Skip this step if you have plastic molds for Popsicle treats.)

In a double boiler, melt chocolate. Add 1 teaspoon SomerSweet and stir well to combine.

With an electric mixer or wire whisk, whip the cream until it starts to become fluffy.

Add the cocoa, 2 teaspoons of Somer-Sweet, and vanilla, and whip until the cream forms soft peaks. Do not overwhip. Fold in the melted chocolate.

Fill the Dixie cups or molds about three-quarters full and place in the freezer until set, about 2 hours.

Put a Popsicle stick in the center of the Fudgysicle and twist to release from the cup. Peel off plastic wrap.

Note
For an even more indulgent treat, make Chocolate Chip Fudgysicles by adding finely chopped-up chocolate to the mixture before pouring into the molds.

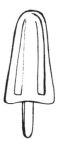

Raspberry Soufflé

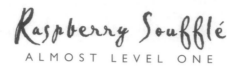

ALMOST LEVEL ONE

SERVES 10

I love soufflés, especially this one, which is virtually free of sugar. Don't be intimidated by a soufflé. It is simply a matter of blending the base (sugarless raspberry jam, and egg yolks with a little sweetener) with the whipped egg whites, and baking them in their individual cups in a roasting pan filled with hot water. They will rise and be beautiful. You can make the base ahead of time and whip the egg whites at the last minute. Try it, you'll like it. This is one of Alan's most often requested desserts.

Butter for greasing the soufflé dishes
4 teaspoons SomerSweet (or 2 teaspoons
　saccharin)
5 eggs, separated
1½ cups sugarless raspberry jam

Whipped cream for garnish

EQUIPMENT
10 (5-ounce) soufflé dishes (ramekins)

Preheat oven to 450 degrees.

Butter the soufflé dishes. Place them in the freezer for 5 minutes. Then butter them again and sprinkle with 1 teaspoon Somer-Sweet (or ½ teaspoon saccharin). Tap out the excess. Store the dishes in the freezer until you are ready to use them.

Beat the egg whites at medium speed until frothy. Then increase the speed to high and beat them until stiff peaks form, adding 2 teaspoons SomerSweet (or 1 teaspoon saccharin). Beat the egg yolks with 1 more teaspoon of SomerSweet (or ½ teaspoon saccharin) until thick and light-colored. Add the raspberry jam. Gently fold the egg whites into the egg yolk mixture.

Fill each dish three-quarters full, and set them in a roasting pan with 1 inch of hot water. Place the roasting pan over low heat on top of the stove. After 1 minute, remove the molds from the water and place them directly on a rack in the center of the oven. Bake for 10 minutes, or until the soufflés are about 2 inches above the top of the mold. Sprinkle with a tiny dusting of SomerSweet and serve immediately with whipped cream.

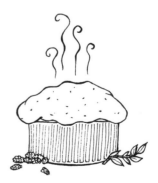

Light Chocolate Mousse

PRO/FATS—ALMOST LEVEL ONE

SERVES 6–8

I love to keep this light treat in the refrigerator. I have a little spoonful when I want something sweet.

2 cups heavy cream, well chilled
3 tablespoons unsweetened cocoa powder
3 teaspoons SomerSweet (or 2 teaspoons saccharin)

2 teaspoons pure vanilla extract

With an electric mixer or wire whisk, whip the cream until it starts to become fluffy.

Add the cocoa, SomerSweet, and vanilla and whip until the cream forms soft peaks. Do not overwhip.

Serve immediately, or chill in the refrigerator.

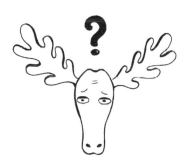

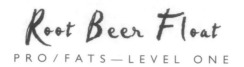

Root Beer Float

MAKES 2

I have a friend named Matt who started Somersizing and lost 18 pounds in the first month! He gave me the recipe for this amazing root beer float. You can make it the traditional way with my sugarless Vanilla Bean Ice Cream. Or you can make it Matt's quick and easy way with a glass full of crushed ice, a splash of heavy cream, and diet root beer. Get ready for a frothy root beer float mustache!

TRADITIONAL RECIPE

2 scoops Vanilla Bean Ice Cream (p. 250)
1 can diet root beer

Chill 2 tall soda glasses in the freezer. Place a generous scoop of vanilla ice cream in each glass. Slowly pour the root beer over the top.

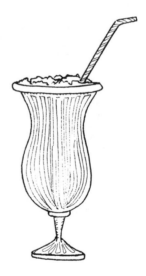

MATT'S RECIPE

Crushed ice
About ½ cup heavy cream
1 can diet root beer

Chill 2 tall soda glasses in the freezer. Fill each glass with crushed ice cubes. Add about ¼ cup cream, then slowly pour in the root beer.

Black-and-White Baked Alaska

ALMOST LEVEL TWO

SERVES 12

I am so excited to bring back this classic recipe from my childhood. It dawned on me one day that using SomerSweet to make the ice cream and the meringue would make it a Level One dessert, yet fit to serve at the most elaborate and elegant dinner party. I have chosen to serve this for my Christmas dinner this year, and no one will realize that eating something so scrumptious is not fattening. The only imbalance in this entire dessert is the chocolate in the ice cream. There are a lot of steps, with a base of meringue, then a layer of vanilla ice cream, a layer of chocolate ice cream, and the beautiful meringue exterior. I'm sure you will agree it is worth the work when you taste your first mouthful and realize that this seemingly sinful dessert is not going to put an ounce of fat on you.

10 large egg whites
2½ tablespoons SomerSweet (or 4
   teaspoons saccharin)

1¼ teaspoons cream of tartar
1 pint Dark Chocolate Ice Cream (p. 251)
2 pints Vanilla Bean Ice Cream (p. 250)

Heat oven to 250 degrees.

The first thing you are going to do is make a meringue base. You will need a pastry bag, parchment paper, and an 8-inch metal bowl.

Place a sheet of parchment paper on a baking sheet. Using an 8-inch metal bowl as your guide, draw a circle on the parchment paper as your pattern for the meringues. (You will also use this bowl later to mold the ice cream.)

To make the meringue, beat 2 egg whites with an electric mixer and slowly add 1½ teaspoons of the SomerSweet and 1 teaspoon cream of tartar. Whip until egg whites are stiff and shiny, about 5 minutes.

Fill the pastry bag with the egg whites

and squeeze out the meringue in a spiral starting at the center of the pattern. Squeeze around and around until the base is the same size as drawn circle.

Place the meringue circle in the preheated oven (still on the sheet of parchment paper) for 50 to 60 minutes, or until it is dry. Do not let it brown. Remove from oven and let it cool completely.

While meringue is baking, line the metal bowl with plastic wrap so the plastic hangs over the edges. Press the chocolate ice cream against the sides of the bowl, leaving a well in the center (you will fill this later with vanilla ice cream), and press to make it smooth. Fold the plastic wrap to cover the top and freeze till hard, about 3 minutes.

When chocolate ice cream has hardened, fill the well with vanilla ice cream. Press to make a smooth top. Cover again with plastic wrap and return to the freezer. Increase oven temperature to 450 degrees.

Now prepare the meringue for the outside layer. Whip the remaining 8 egg whites with 2 tablespoons SomerSweet and ¼ teaspoon of cream of tartar until the whites are very stiff and shiny, about 7–8 minutes.

To assemble, place the cooked meringue disk on an ovenproof serving dish. Unmold frozen ice cream on top of the disk. Spoon the whipped meringue all over the top of the ice cream and swirl it around decoratively with the back of the spoon. (The hills and valleys of the egg whites will brown beautifully.)

Place in oven until top meringue becomes golden brown, 2–4 minutes. Serve immediately or put back into the freezer until ready to serve.

Note

You can place the completely assembled Baked Alaska in the freezer the day before and remove it 1 hour before serving, and it will turn out perfectly. This way you eliminate last-minute worries. Make sure your serving dish is of the type that can go from the oven to the freezer without shattering.

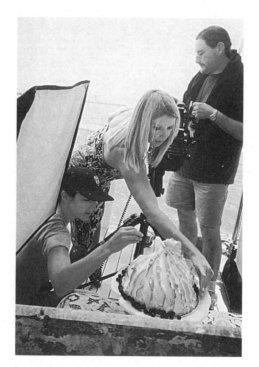

My daughter-in-law, Caroline, myself, and my favorite photographer, Jeff Katz, getting the Baked Alaska ready for the photo shoot.

Chocolate Fondue

LEVEL TWO

SERVES 6–8

The best part of any fondue party is dessert! This Chocolate Fondue is divine with fresh berries.

16 ounces dark chocolate (at least 60% cocoa)
2 cups heavy cream

1 basket fresh strawberries
1 basket fresh blackberries
1 basket fresh raspberries

Chop the chocolate into small pieces and place in a heatproof bowl. Heat the cream in a small saucepan just until it reaches a boil. Add the hot cream to the chocolate.

Stir with a wooden spoon until the chocolate is melted through.

Transfer immediately to a fondue pot and serve with fresh berries.

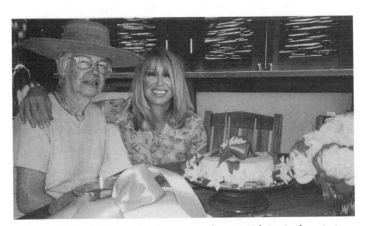

Sugarless Cheesecake for my Aunt Helen's birthday. She is diabetic and loves that she can eat this without worrying.

Molten Chocolate Cakes

LEVEL TWO

SERVES 6

Sinful, decadent, rich, and delicious. These divine little cakes ooze with melted chocolate in the center.

9 ounces dark chocolate (at least 60% cocoa)

11 tablespoons unsalted butter plus some for custard cups

3 large eggs

3 large egg yolks

4 teaspoons SomerSweet (or 2 teaspoons saccharin)

¼ cup whole wheat pastry flour

Whipped cream for garnish

Fresh raspberries for garnish

Preheat oven to 325 degrees.

Butter 6 small glass custard cups, about 3–4 ounces.

In a double boiler, heat 6 ounces of chocolate and the butter over 3 inches of simmering water, until melted.

With the whisk attachment on the mixer, mix eggs, yolks, and SomerSweet or saccharin until pale and thick, about 10 minutes. Add flour and melted chocolate and mix for 5 more minutes.

Pour batter into custard cups until almost half full. Place ½ ounce of chopped choco-late in the center of the batter in each cup, then pour more batter on top, dividing the batter equally among the 6 cups.

Place the cups in the oven and bake for about 12 minutes, until sides seem stiff but center jiggles when you touch.

Cool for a few minutes. Slide knife around sides of cups to make sure the cake will slide out when flipped over. Invert each onto a plate and remove custard cup. Prick the center with a fork and this fabulous chocolate oozes out like lava. Serve with whipped cream and fresh raspberries.

Panna Cotta (Italian Custard)

SERVES 4

This beautiful custard makes me smile. It will make your taste buds sing.

2 teaspoons unflavored gelatin
1½ cups heavy cream
½ teaspoon SomerSweet (or ¼ teaspoon
   saccharin)

½ teaspoon vanilla extract
1 or 2 drops yellow food coloring
2 cups mixed fresh berries, such as
   raspberries, blueberries, and blackberries

In a medium saucepan, sprinkle gelatin over cream. Let stand 2 minutes.

Put the saucepan over medium heat and add SomerSweet to the cream and gelatin. Cook, stirring to dissolve SomerSweet, until small bubbles appear around edges of pan. Add vanilla and food coloring.

Divide mixture among four 4-ounce ramekins. Cover and refrigerate for 4 hours or overnight.

Fill a small bowl with warm water and dip molds into warm water, but do not fully submerge. Run the tip of a knife around the edge to loosen panna cotta. Invert each mold onto a dessert plate. Garnish with berries and serve immediately.

Parisian Hot Chocolate

LEVEL TWO

SERVES 4

Curl up with a mug by the fire and sip this hot chocolate. It's almost guilt free! The cocoa powder creates a minor imbalance, but otherwise it's all Level One. And because it's sweetened with Somer-Sweet, you don't have to worry about all the sugar you find in regular hot chocolate. This is how they make it in Paris, with a touch of cinnamon and nutmeg.

4 cups heavy cream
1 cup water
1 tablespoon plus 1 teaspoon vanilla extract
$\frac{1}{2}$ cup plus 1 tablespoon unsweetened
   cocoa powder

2 tablespoons plus 2 teaspoons SomerSweet
   (or 2 teaspoons saccharin)
$\frac{1}{4}$ teaspoon cinnamon
$\frac{1}{4}$ teaspoon nutmeg
Whipped cream for garnish (optional)

Combine and stir all ingredients except whipped cream in a heavy bottomed saucepan. Whisk constantly over medium heat until hot but not boiling. Pour into mugs and top with whipped cream if desired.

Cherry Clafouti

SERVES 8

This is a great dessert to make during the summer months when cherries are in season, especially if you can get the Queen Anne cherries. They are lighter in color and usually sweeter. Be sure to leave the pits in. For some reason, the flavor intensifies and literally pops in your mouth. In addition, the cherries won't sink, and this is the way it is traditionally done in France. If fresh cherries are not available, frozen cherries are delicious. This dessert is Level Two because of the flour, but it will not create too much of an imbalance because the flour is whole wheat, the amount is very small, and it is sweetened with SomerSweet.

1½ pounds fresh cherries (or 2 pounds
    frozen cherries)
Butter for the baking dish
2 eggs
1 egg yolk
2 teaspoons SomerSweet, plus some for
    dusting (or 1 teaspoon saccharin)

5 tablespoons butter, melted
⅔ cup whole wheat pastry flour
1 cup heavy cream
Crème fraîche (optional)

Preheat oven to 400 degrees.

Wash, dry, and destem the cherries.

Butter an ovenproof decorative baking dish (I use a porcelain quiche baking dish).

Place the cherries in the baking dish. Combine the eggs and the yolk in a bowl, add the SomerSweet, and whisk in the melted butter. Sift in the flour and mix well. Then mix in the cream and continue beating until the batter is smooth. Pour over the cherries.

Bake for 40 minutes, until golden brown. Remove from oven and dust lightly with a little more SomerSweet.

Serve lukewarm from the baking dish, with crème fraîche if desired.

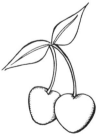

Chocolate Truffles

LEVEL TWO

MAKES ABOUT 30 (1-OUNCE) TRUFFLES

Thank God for my SomerSweet; it makes sinful treats, like this, sugar free without the harmful effects of artificial sweeteners. And if you don't have the time to make these, you can buy a box already prepared at SuzanneSomers.com!

6 ounces unsweetened chocolate, chopped
1½ cups heavy cream
½ teaspoon orange extract
2 tablespoons plus ½ teaspoon
　　SomerSweet (or 2 teaspoons saccharin)

Unsweetened cocoa powder for dusting
6 ounces chopped dark chocolate, at least
　　60% cocoa (optional)

Place chopped chocolate in the bowl of a food processor.

Heat cream in a saucepan over medium heat until small bubbles appear around the edge. Pour cream over chocolate and allow to stand for 30 seconds. Blend until mixture is smooth. Add orange extract and Somer-Sweet. Transfer mixture to a shallow dish and refrigerate until hard, at least 1 hour.

Using a 1-ounce portion scoop or a tablespoon, scoop out balls of chocolate and place on a baking sheet. Place sheet in the refrigerator for about 30 minutes.

When chilled, roll each truffle in the palm of your hand into a perfect round.

Drop truffles into cocoa powder to finish.

Store truffles refrigerated in an airtight container.

For a slightly more indulgent treat, after coating the truffles in cocoa powder, coat them in dark chocolate. Melt 6 ounces chopped dark chocolate (at least 60% cocoa) in a double boiler until smooth. Using a skewer or toothpick, spear each truffle and dip into the melted chocolate. Allow the excess coating to drip off, and use a second toothpick to push the truffle onto a sheet pan lined with wax or parchment paper. Refrigerate until coating has hardened.

Appendix

When I first discovered this remarkable way of eating I was determined to find medical research to make sure my program was not only effective, but safe. If raised insulin levels are responsible for weight, increased cholesterol, hypertension, heart disease, and certain types of cancer, why aren't doctors telling us to worry about our sugar intake?

Surprisingly, finding the medical backup was not difficult at all. The effects of high insulin levels (resulting from overeating sugar/carbohydrates/caffeine or from stress) and their relationship to weight gain, abnormal cholesterol levels, coronary heart disease, and Type II diabetes have been documented in numerous medical studies that span more than thirty years! This is hardly new information.

Specifically, I want to share three articles, linking high insulin levels to these diseases. The first is from *The New England Journal of Medicine.* "Risk Factors for Coronary Artery Disease in Healthy Persons with Hyperinsulinemia and Normal Glucose Tolerance" (March 16, 1989) concluded that healthy persons with hyperinsulinemia and normal glucose levels are at higher risk for coronary artery disease, as compared with a well-matched group of healthy subjects with normal insulin levels.

The second article is from *Diabetes Care,* "Insulin Resistance: A Multifaceted Syndrome Responsible for NIDDM, Obesity, Hypertension, Dyslipidemia, and Atherosclerotic Cardiovascular Disease" (Vol. 14, no. 3, March 1991). I'll share with you a passage from the summary:

Much evidence has begun to accumulate that chronic day-long hyperinsulinemia is associated with the development of hypertension [high blood pressure], hyperlipidemia [high cholesterol and triglycerides], and atherosclerosis [clogged arteries]. In a sense, insulin

resistance can be viewed as a large iceberg submerged just below the surface of the water. The physician recognizes only the tip of the iceberg—diabetes, obesity, hypertension, hypertriglyceridemia, diminished HDL-chol, and atherosclerosis—which extrude above the surface, and complete insulin resistance may be missed.

The third article from *Diabetes Care,* "Insulin and Atheroma: A 20-Year Perspective" (Vol. 13, no. 6, June 1990), outlines the research on the subject of insulin for the last twenty years. This comprehensive study concludes:

The fact that hyperinsulinemia has been shown to have an independent predictive correlation with cardiovascular disease and that insulin has biological actions on arterial tissue, lipid metabolism, and renal sodium handling suggest that the primary abnormality may be hyperinsulinemia due to insulin resistance.

Check out these articles for yourself.

Reference Guide

Here is a complete list of all the foods available in each of the categories:

PRO/FATS

CHEESE
American
asiago
Babybel
bel paese
blue
Bonbel
Brie
buffalo mozzarella
Camembert
cheddar
Colby
cream cheese
farmer
feta
fontina
goat
gouda

Gruyère
Havarti
hoop
Jarlsberg
Limburger
mascarpone
Monterey jack
mozzarella
Muenster
Parmesan
pecorino
provolone
queso blanco
ricotta
Romano
Roquefort
string
Swiss

OTHER DAIRY
PRODUCTS
butter
cream
eggs
margarine
mayonnaise
sour cream

FISH
anchovy
bass
bluefish
bonito
burbot
carp
catfish
cod

eel
flatfish
flounder
gefilte fish
grouper
haddock
halibut
herring
mackerel
mahi-mahi
monkfish
ocean perch
orange roughy
pollack
pompano
red snapper
sablefish
salmon

sardine
sea bass
shark
smelt
snapper
sole
sturgeon
swordfish
trout
tuna
turbot
whitefish
wolf fish
yellowtail

MEAT
bacon
Canadian bacon
beef
bratwurst
bologna
capocollo
cold cuts
frog's legs
ham
hot dogs
lamb
pastrami
pepperoni
pork
prosciutto
rabbit
salami

sausage
veal
venison

OILS
chili oil
olive oil
peanut oil
safflower oil
sesame oil
vegetable oil

POULTRY
capon
chicken
Cornish game hen
duck
goose
guinea hen

pheasant
quail
squab
turkey

SEAFOOD
abalone
caviar
clams
crab
crayfish
lobster
mussels
octopus
scallops
shrimp
squid

CARBOS

BEANS
adzuki beans
anasazi beans
black beans
black-eyed peas
cannellini beans
fava beans
garbanzo beans
great northern
    beans
green peas
kidney beans
lentils
lima beans
mung beans
navy beans
pinto beans

red beans
split peas
white beans

BREADS,
BAGELS,
CRACKERS,
HOT CEREALS,
COLD CEREALS,
OR PASTA MADE
FROM WHOLE
GRAINS
amaranth
barley
bran
brown rice
buckwheat

durum wheat
farina
kamut
millet
oats
pumpernickel
rye
spelt
wheat

TABBOULEH

WHEAT GERM

PHYLLO DOUGH

NONFAT DAIRY
PRODUCTS
    nonfat cottage
        cheese
    nonfat milk
    nonfat rice milk
    nonfat ricotta
        cheese
    nonfat sour
        cream
    nonfat soy milk
    nonfat yogurt

RICE
    brown rice
    brown rice cakes
    wild rice

VEGGIES

alfalfa sprouts
artichoke
arugula
asparagus
bamboo shouts
basil
bean sprouts
beet greens
bok choy
broccoli
brussels sprouts
cabbage
cauliflower
celery
chervil
chicory greens
chives
cilantro
clover sprouts
collard greens
crookneck squash

cucumber
daikon
dandelion greens
dill weed
eggplant
endive
escarole
fennel
garlic
ginger
green beans
horseradish
jicama
kale
kohlrabi
leeks
lettuce
  Boston or bibb
  frisée
  iceberg
  limestone

  red oak
  romaine
mushrooms
mustard greens
okra
onion
parsley
peppers
  bell peppers
  cherry peppers
  chili peppers
  peperoncini
  piccalilli
pickles (except sweet)
purslane
radicchio
radish
rhubarb
rosemary
sage
salsify

sauerkraut
scallions
shallots
snow peas
spinach
sugar snap peas
Swiss chard
tarragon
thyme
tomatillo
tomato
tomato (green)
turnip
turnip greens
water chestnut
watercress
wax beans
yard-long beans
yellow beans
yucca
zucchini

FRUIT

apples
apricots
Asian pear
berries
  blackberry
  blueberry
  boysenberry
  cranberry
  currant
  elderberry
  gooseberry
  mulberry
  ollalaberry
  raspberry

  strawberry
cherimoya
cherry
crabapple
fig
grapefruit
grapes
guava
kiwi
kumquat
lemon
lime
loquat
lychee

mangoes
mandarin oranges
melons
  cantaloupe
  casaba
  Crenshaw
  honeydew
  orange flesh
  sharlyn
watermelon
nectarines
oranges
papaya
passion fruit

peaches
pears
persimmon
pineapple
plums
pomegranate
prickly pear
pommelo
quince
star fruit
tamarind
tangerine

YOUR ONE-PAGE REFERENCE GUIDE

For the first few days or weeks on the program, you might want to make a copy of this page and slip it into your purse or wallet. Somersizing will soon become second nature to you, but this summary will help remind you of the plan until you no longer need it for reference.

1. Eliminate all Funky Foods.
2. Eat Fruits alone, on an empty stomach.
3. Eat Proteins/Fats with Veggies.
4. Eat Carbos with Veggies and no fat.
5. Keep Proteins/Fats separate from Carbos.
6. Wait three hours between meals if switching from a Proteins/Fats meal to a Carbos meal, or vice versa.
7. Do not skip meals. Eat three meals a day, and eat until you feel satisfied and comfortably full.

PROTEINS AND FATS

Butter	Mayonnaise
Cheese	Meat
Cream	Oil
Eggs	Poultry
Fish	Sour cream

VEGGIES

Asparagus	Green beans
Broccoli	Lettuce
Cauliflower	Mushrooms
Celery	Spinach
Cucumber	Tomato
Eggplant	Zucchini

CARBOS

Beans	Whole-grain
Mustard	breads, cereals,
Nonfat milk	pastas
products	Nonfat soy milk

FRUITS

Apples	Oranges
Berries	Papaya
Grapes	Peaches
Mangoes	Pears
Melons	Plums
Nectarines	

Eliminate Funky Foods

SUGAR

Beets	Maple syrup
Carrots	Molasses
Corn syrup	Sugar
Honey	

STARCHES

Bananas	Potatoes
Corn	Sweet potatoes
Pasta made from	White flour
semolina or	White rice
white flour	Winter squashes
Popcorn	(acorn, butternut)

COMBO PROTEINS/FATS AND CARBOS

Avocados	Nuts
Buttermilk	Olives
Coconuts	Tofu
Liver	
Low-fat or	
whole milk	

CAFFEINE AND ALCOHOL

Alcoholic beverages
Caffeinated coffees, teas, and sodas
Cocoa (including unsweetened cocoa)

Bibliography

Anderson, K. M., W. P. Castelli, and D. Levy. "Cholesterol and Mortality: 30 Years of Follow-up from the Framingham Study," *JAMA* 257(1987): 2176–80.

Applegate, Liz. "Fats as Fuel? A Little More Fat in Your Diet May Help You on Your Next Run," *Runner's World* 29, no. 6 (June 1994): 24.

Atkins, Robert C. "Artificial Sugar: A Sweet and Dangerous Lure," *Dr. Atkins' Health Revelations* (April 1994): 1.

Brown, David. "Linkage of Breast Cancer, Dietary Fat Is Discounted," *The Washington Post* 119, no. 65 (February 8, 1996): A5 col 1.

Carlson, L. A., L. E. Bottiger, and P. E. Anfeldt. "Risk Factors for Myocardial Infarction in the Stockholm Prospective Study: A 14-year Follow-up Focusing on the Role of Plasma Triglycerides and Cholesterol," *Acta Med Scand* 206 (1979): 351–60.

Clark, Nancy. "Fat and Fiction: Dispelling the Myths About Fat in a Healthy Diet," *American Fitness* 15, no. 3 (May–June 1997): 59.

DeFronzo, R. A. "Insulin Secretion, Insulin Resistance, and Obesity." *Int J Obes* 6 (Suppl. 1) (1982): 72–82.

DeFronzo, R. A., and E. Ferrannini. "Insulin Resistance: A Multifaceted Syndrome Responsible for NIDDM, Obesity, Hypertension, Dyslipemia, and Atherosclerotic Cardiovascular Disease," *Diabetes Care* 14, no. 3 (March 1991): 173.

Fackelmann, K. "Hidden Hazards: Do High Blood Insulin Levels Foretell Heart Disease?" *Science News* 136 (September 16, 1989): 184.

Fontbonne, A. "Why Can High Insulin Levels Indicate a Risk Factor for Coronary Heart Disease?" *Diabetologia* 37 (1994): 953–55.

Grundy, Scott M. "Cholesterol and Coronary Disease," *JAMA* 256 (1986): 2849–58.

———. "Fats and Oil Consumption to Combat Metabolic Complications and Obesity," *American Journal of Clinical Nutrition* 67, no. 3 (March 1998): 5275.

Howe, Maggy. "Good Fats, Bad Fats," *Country Living* 21, no. 1 (January 1998): 50.

Jenkins, J. A., et al. "Starchy Foods and Glycemic Index," *Diabetes Care* 11, no. 2 (February 1998): 149.

Modann, M., H. Halkin, S. Almog, et al. "Hyperinsulinemia: A Link Between Hypertension, Obesity, and Glucose Intolerance," *J Clin Invest* 75 (1985): 809–17.

Page, Douglas. "Give Fat a Break," *Muscle and Fitness* 58, no. 5 (May 1997): 58.

Pollare, T., H. Lithell, and C. Berne. "Insulin Resistance Is a Characteristic Feature of Primary Hypertension Independent of Obesity," *Metabolism* 39 (1990): 167–74.

Raloff, Janet. "High Fat Diets Help Athletes Perform," *Science News* 149, no. 18 (May 4, 1996): 287.

Reaven, G. M. "Banting Lecture: Role of Insulin Resistance in Human Disease," *Diabetes* 37 (1988): 1595–1607.

Reaven, G. M., C. B. Hollenbeck, and Y-DI Chen. "Relationship Between Glucose Tolerance, Insulin Secretion, and Insulin Action in Non-Obese Individuals with Varying Degrees of Glucose Tolerance," *Diabetologia* 32 (1989): 52–55.

Reppert, Bertha, and Sharon Mikkelson. "Stevia (Stevia rebaudiana 'honeyleaf')," *American Health and Herbs* (1998): 1–7.

Schechter, Steven. "Fat Intake Can Boost Weight Loss, if We Are Selective About Our Choices," *Better Nutrition* 59, no. 6 (June 1997): 26.

Schwarzbein, Diana, and Nancy Deville. *The Schwarzbein Principle.* Calif.: Health Communications, Inc., 1999.

Shapiro, Laura. "In Sugar We Trust," *Newsweek* (July 13, 1998): 72.

Sowers, J. R., M. Nyby, N. Stern, F. Beck, S. Baron, R. Catania, and N. Vlachis. "Blood Pressure and Hormone Changes Associated with Weight Reduction in the Obese," *Hypertension* 4 (1982): 686–91.

Stout, Robert W. "Insulin and Atheroma Twenty Year Perspective." *Diabetes Care* 13, no. 6 (June 1990): 631.

Wingard, D. L., E. L. Barrett-Connor, and A. Ferrara. "Is Insulin Really a Heart Disease Risk Factor?" *Diabetes Care* 18 (1995): 1299–1304.

Zavaroni, I., et al. "Risk Factors for Coronary Artery Disease in Healthy Persons with Hyperinsulinemia and Normal Glucose Tolerance," *NEJM* 320 (March 16, 1989): 702.

Index

Addictions, 69
Adrenaline, xix, 76
Aging, accelerated metabolic, 58
Aging process, xviii, 32, 34, 42, 54
Alcohol, 75
Alkalize or Die (Baroody), 79
Amino acids, 76–77
Andy's Feta and Herb Frittata, 139
Antipasto, Grilled Vegetable, 191
Artichoke Pesto, 154
Artichokes, Grilled, 194
Artificial sweeteners, 117
Arugula:
  Pan-Fried Garlic Lemon Shrimp with Zucchini Pesto Noodles and, 214
  and Parmesan Salad, 174
Asparagus, 79
  with Butter and Parmesan, 195
  Chicken Meatball Soup, 163

Aspartame, 35, 73
Atkins, Robert C., 30, 32

Baby Back Pork Ribs, 230
Bad combo foods, 75
Baked Alaska, Black-and-White, 256–57
Balanced diet, importance of, xvii–xviii
Balsamic Syrup, Chicken with Goat Cheese and, 224
Baroody, Theodore A., 79
Basil Pesto, 155
Bean(s), 98, 120
  Black, Vegetable Chili, 204–5
  Chinese Long, 198
  Green, and Hearts of Palm Salad, 176
  Red, and Parsley Salad, 179
  White, Salad with Sage and Thyme, 180
Beef:
  Carne Asada de Perez, 245

Florentine Steak, 247
  Ground, Egg Crêpes with Filling of, 134
  Hamburgers, 241
  Jalapeño Chili, 240–41
  Meatballs, 239
  Meat Fondue, 237
  Meat Sauce, 238
  Peppered Filet with Bourbon Sauce, 244
  Prime Rib au Jus with Garlic Crust, 246–47
  Stew, 242
  Stir-Fry, 243
  Swiss Cheese Fondue, 236
Beverages, *see* Drinks
Black-and-White Baked Alaska, 256–57
Black Bean Vegetable Chili, 204–5
Blood sugar, 21, 22, 23, 24, 48
Blue Cheese Dip, 146
  Buffalo Wings with, 219
Borage oil, 32
Bourbon Sauce, 244

Breads:
 Multigrain, 184
 Parmesan Croutons, 171
 Rye, 183
 Somersize Zucchini
  Muffins, 128
 whole-grain, 97–98, 116
 Whole Wheat, 182
Breakfast meals:
 analysis of, 50–51
 importance of, 121
 Level One, 83–86
 Level Two, 111–12
Breakfast recipes, 127–40
 Andy's Feta and Herb Frit-
  tata, 139
 Creamy Parmesan Sauce,
  135
 Dawn's Deviled Eggs, 129
 Egg Crêpes, 131
 Egg Crêpes with Ground
  Beef Filling, 134
 Egg Crêpes with Spinach
  and Ricotta Filling, 133
 Egg Crêpes with Wild
  Mushroom Filling, 132
 Eggs Baked in Tomatoes in
  Red Peppers, 136
 Grilled Onion Frittata, 137
 Mexican Omelette, 140
 Mozzarella Marinara, 130
 Somersize Zucchini
  Muffins, 128
 Spinach Parmesan Frittata,
  138
Broccoli, Spicy, 202
Broth:
 Chicken, Egg Crêpe Noo-
  dles in, 162
 Quick Chicken, 161
Brunch, see Breakfast recipes
Buffalo Wings with Blue
 Cheese Dip, 219
Burgers:
 Hamburgers, 241
 Lamburgers, 231
 Lemony Chicken, 221
Buttermilk, 116
Butter Sauce, Red Wine, 157

Caesar Salad, 173
 Dressing, 173
 Parmesan Bowls with, 172
Caffeine, 75, 76, 120
Cakes, Molten Chocolate, 259
Calories, 7–13
 cutting down on, 7–10
 daily intake of, 8
 and survival instinct, 8–10
 and weight, 19
Canned goods, 99–100
Caramelized Fennel, 196
Carbohydrate Addict's Diet,
  17
Carbohydrates, 10, 77, 268
 complex, 23, 24
 cravings for, 51–52, 116
 and food combining, 46
 as fuel, 25
 Glycemic Index for, 81
 low-carb diet plans, 3
 low-starch, 46–47
 in the morning, 41, 120
 Pro/Fats and, 105–7, 270
 proteins and fats separated
  from, 1, 27
 in refined form, 23
 simple, 23
 sources of, 21
 veggies as, 78
Carne Asada de Perez, 245
Castelli, William, 31
Catfish, Crispy Fried, with
  Ginger Chips, 212
Celery root, 123
 Green Chili Puree, 190
Cells, healthy, 32–35
Cereals, 98, 116, 118
Cheating, 103–4

Cheese Fondue, Swiss, 236
Chemicals, in body, xviii–xix,
  34
Cherry Clafouti, 262
Chewing gum, 123
Chicken:
 Breasts with Sage, 223
 Buffalo Wings with Blue
  Cheese Dip, 219
 Cacciatore, 225
 Flattened, 222
 with Goat Cheese and Bal-
  samic Syrup, 224
 Lemony Burgers, 221
 Meatball Asparagus Soup,
  163
 Quick Broth, 161
 Southern Country Fried,
  Salad, 178
 Swiss Cheese Fondue, 236
Children, Somersizing for,
  60–67
Chili:
 Black Bean Vegetable, 204–5
 Jalapeño, 240–41
Chinese food, 122
Chinese Long Beans, 198
Chips, Parmesan, 170
Chocolate, 110, 122
 Chip Fudgysicles, 252
 Dark, Ice Cream, 251
 Fondue, 258
 Light Mousse, 254
 Molten, Cakes, 259
 Parisian Hot, 261
 Sugarless Fudgysicles, 252
 Truffles, 263
Cholecystokinin (CCK), 39
Cholesterol, 39–41
 body's manufacture of, 41
 as building block, 40
 HDL (good), 41
 and hormonal imbalance, 22
 and insulin resistance, 28
 research on, 42–43

and sugar, 2
and trans fats, 30
Chunky Jalapeño Guacamole, 150
Clafouti, Cherry, 262
Clam Bake!, 210–11
Comfort foods, 20, 76, 77
Commitment, 70
Complex carbohydrates, 23, 24
Control, 68–70, 109–10
Conversion chart, 282
Cool Mocha Coolers, 144
Crab Bake!, 210–11
Crab Dip, Hot, 147
Cream of Green Chili Soup, 160
Creamy Parmesan Sauce, 135
Creamy Shallot Sauce, Pork Chops with, 228
Crêpes, Egg, 131
    with Ground Beef Filling, 134
    Noodles in Chicken Broth, 162
    with Spinach and Ricotta Filling, 133
    with Wild Mushroom Filling, 132
Crispy Fried Catfish with Ginger Chips, 212
Croutons, Parmesan, 171
Custard, Savory, Rosemary-Infused, with Tomato Mushroom Sauce, 192–93
Custard, Italian (Panna Cotta), 260

Dairy products, 82, 98, 117, 119–20, 122
Dark Chocolate Ice Cream, 251
Dawn's Deviled Eggs, 129

Deep-Fried Turkey with Fried Onions and Herbs, 220
Desserts, 249–63
    Black-and-White Baked Alaska, 256–57
    Cherry Clafouti, 262
    Chocolate Chip Fudgysicles, 252
    Chocolate Fondue, 258
    Chocolate Truffles, 263
    Dark Chocolate Ice Cream, 251
    Light Chocolate Mousse, 254
    Molten Chocolate Cakes, 259
    Panna Cotta (Italian Custard), 260
    Parisian Hot Chocolate, 261
    Raspberry Soufflé, 253
    Root Beer Float, 255
    Sugarless Fudgysicles, 252
    Vanilla Bean Ice Cream, 250
Deviled Eggs, Dawn's, 129
Diabetes, 23, 33, 123, 265–66
Diet drinks, 34–35
Diets, 14–19
    Carbohydrate Addict, 17
    Dr. Atkins' Revolution, 15
    low-fat, 37
    Protein Power, 15, 17
    Somersize, 18–19
    Sugar Busters, 18
    The Zone, 17–18
Dining out, 95–96, 118
Dinners:
    Level One, 86–88
    Level Two, 111–12
Dips:
    Artichoke Pesto, 154
    Blue Cheese, 146
    Hot Crab, 147
    Spinach, 148
Dr. Atkins' Diet Revolution, 15

Drinks, 100, 117–18, 141–44
    Cool Mocha Coolers, 144
    diet, 34–35
    Fresh Mint Tea, 142
    Parisian Hot Chocolate, 261
    Rich Mocha Coolers, 143
    Root Beer Float, 255

Eat Great, Lose Weight (Somers), 2, 13, 26, 110
Eating disorders, 64
Eggplant Parmesan, 207
Eggs, 31, 98, 119
    Andy's Feta and Herb Frittata, 139
    Baked in Tomatoes and Red Peppers, 136
    Crêpe Noodles in Chicken Broth, 162
    Crêpes, 131
    Crêpes with Ground Beef Filling, 134
    Crêpes with Spinach and Ricotta Filling, 133
    Crêpes with Wild Mushroom Filling, 132
    Dawn's Deviled, 129
    Grilled Onion Frittata, 137
    Mexican Omelette, 140
    Spinach Parmesan Frittata, 138
    Stracciatella Soup, 166
Equivalents for ingredients, 282
Estradiol, xviii, xix, 56
Estrogen, 56, 59
Exercise, 101–2

Fat-free foods, 23–24, 30, 49, 116
Fats, 26–35
    and hormones, 32
    research on, 13, 42–43
    saturated vs. unsaturated, 29

separation from carbohy-
drates, 1, 27
trans, 29–30
and weight, 19
as your friend, 28–32, 36,
39, 40, 77
Fennel:
with Butter and Parmesan
Cheese, 197
Caramelized, 196
Feta and Herb Frittata, Andy's,
139
Fiber, 23, 47
Fish and shellfish, 209–16
Clam Bake! Mussel Bake!
Crab Bake! Lobster Bake!,
210–11
Crispy Fried Catfish with
Ginger Chips, 212
Grilled Ginger Shrimp on
Skewers, 213
Orange Roughy with
Mushroom Stuffing, 215
Pan-Fried Garlic Lemon
Shrimp with Zucchini
Pesto Noodles and
Arugula, 214
Pan-Fried Petrale Sole with
Lemon, Butter, and
Caper Sauce, 216
Red Hot Singing Scallops,
211
Flattened Chicken, 222
Florentine Steak, 247
Fondue:
Chocolate, 258
Meat, 237
Pesto, with Sausages, 218
Swiss Cheese, 236
Food categories, 10–11, 75
combining, 11–12, 46–52
reference guide, 267–70
Food cravings, 51–52, 116
Food Pyramid, USDA, 36
Free foods, 80–81
Free radicals, 34, 35

Fresh Mint Tea, 142
Frittatas:
Andy's Feta and Herb, 139
Grilled Onion, 137
Spinach Parmesan, 138
Fructose, 73
Fruits, 10, 79–80, 100, 269,
270
dried, 80, 116
guidelines for, 80, 120–21
in Level Two, 107
Fudgysicles, Sugarless, 252
Funky Foods, 11
bad combo foods, 75
caffeine and alcohol, 75
elimination of, 46, 72, 270
in Level Two, 107–9
starches, 74–75
sugars, 72

Garlic Crust, Prime Rib au
Jus with, 246–47
Get Skinny on Fabulous Food
(Somers), 2–3, 13, 26,
28–29, 40, 49, 110
Ginger Chips, Crispy Fried
Catfish with, 212
Gingered Snap Peas, 199
Ginger Shrimp on Skewers,
Grilled, 213
Glucose, 21, 77, 265
Glycemic Index, 81
Glycogen, 8
Goat Cheese, Chicken with
Balsamic Syrup and, 224
Gravy, Roasted Turkey, 158
Green Bean and Hearts of
Palm Salad, 176
Green Chili:
Celery Root Puree, 190
Cream Soup, 160
Green Goddess Dressing, 149
Grilled Artichokes, 194
Grilled Ginger Shrimp on
Skewers, 213

Grilled Marinated Lamb
Chops with Lemon, 233
Grilled Onion Frittata, 137
Grilled Vegetable Antipasto,
191
Guacamole, Chunky Jalapeño,
150
Gum, chewing, 123

Hamburgers, 241
Heart disease:
causes of, 39–41
and insulin resistance, 28,
265
and sugar, 2
Hearts of Palm and Green
Bean Salad, 176
Hearty Mushroom Lasagna,
186
Herbs, 100
HMG-CoA reductase, 40
Hormonal imbalance, xv–xvi,
xvii, 19, 22, 33–34,
53–59
Hormone replacement therapy
(HRT), xvii, xviii–xix,
55–56, 59
Hormones:
and fats, 32
importance of, 53
and metabolism, 42
natural, 56–57
and obesity, 53–54
synthetic, 58
tracking of, xix
Hot Chocolate, Parisian, 261
Hot Crab Dip, 147
Hyperinsulinemia, 23, 265–66

Ice cream, 50, 120
Dark Chocolate, 251
Vanilla Bean, 250
Ingredients, conversion chart,
282

Insulin, 19, 21–22, 265
    and cholesterol, 40
    as fat-storing hormone, 42,
        54
    and fiber, 23
    lowering of, 43
    and pancreas, 22, 23, 24
Insulin resistance, xix, 21, 22,
    28, 34
Israeli Salad, 175
Italian Custard (Panna Cotta),
    260

*J*alapeño:
    Chili, 240–41
    Chunky Guacamole, 150
Jell-O, 115
Juice, 116–17, 122

*K*etchup, 115

*L*amb:
    Baby Chops with Parmesan
        Crusts and Sweet Tomato
        Sauce, 234–35
    Grilled Marinated Chops
        with Lemon, 233
    Lamburgers, 231
    Loin with Tarragon Salsa,
        232
Lasagna, Hearty Mushroom,
    186
Lemonade drinks, 121
Lemon Tarragon Vinaigrette,
    152
Lemony Chicken Burgers, 221
Lettuce, 99
Level One, 11–13, 25, 52,
    83–102
    breakfast, 83–86
    cheating in, 89–91
    commitment to, 91
    Level Two and, 104–5
    lunch and dinner, 86–88
    rhythm in, 88–89

sample week, 93–95
    SomerSweet and, 92–93
Level Two, 103–14
    meal plans, 110–12
Lifestyle:
    of children, 60–61
    and weight gain, 41–42
Light Chocolate Mousse, 254
Liver, 123
Lobster Bake!, 210–11
Lo Han Kuo fruit, 73
Long Beans, Chinese, 198
Lunch and dinner:
    Level One, 86–88
    Level Two, 111–12

*M*argarine, 119
Matt's Recipe for Root Beer
    Float, 255
Mayonnaise, 49, 98–99, 115
Measures, conversion chart,
    282
Meat, 99, 118, 227–47
    Fondue, 237
    Meatballs, 239
    Sauce, 238
    see also specific meats
Medroxyprogesterone acetate,
    xviii
Melt, The, 37, 39
Menopause, xviii, 54–59
Metabolism, 21, 24–25
    and aging process, 34, 42
    inborn errors of, xvi, 25
    and weight gain, 41–42
Mexican Omelette, 140
Middle Eastern Vegetable Stew,
    206
Mint Tea, Fresh, 142
Mirror, standing naked before,
    22
Mocha Coolers, 143–44
Molten Chocolate Cakes, 259
Mousse, Light Chocolate, 254
Mozzarella Marinara, 130

Muffins, Somersize Zucchini,
    128
Multigrain Bread, 184
Mushroom(s):
    Hearty Lasagna, 186
    Portobellos with Bubbling
        Pesto, 200
    Stuffing, Orange Roughy
        with, 215
    Tomato Sauce, 193
    Watercress Soup, 167
    Wild, Egg Crêpes with
        Filling of, 132
Mussel Bake!, 210–11

*N*ew Year celebration, 66–67
Niçoise Salad, 177
Noodles:
    Egg Crêpe, in Chicken
        Broth, 162
    Zucchini, 203
    Zucchini Pesto, Pan-Fried
        Garlic Lemon Shrimp
        with Arugula and, 214
Nursing women, 45
Nuts, 121

*O*besity, 23, 26, 53–54, 61
Oil, 99, 115, 117, 119
Olestra, 24
Omega-3 and omega-6 fatty
    acids, 31, 32
Omelette, Mexican, 140
Onion(s):
    Fried, Deep-Fried Turkey
        with Herbs and, 220
    Grilled Frittata, 137
Orange Roughy with Mush-
    room Stuffing, 215
Osteoporosis, 57

*P*ancreas, function of, 21, 22,
    23, 24

Pan-Fried Garlic Lemon
    Shrimp with Zucchini
    Pesto Noodles and
    Arugula, 214
Pan-Fried Petrale Sole with
    Lemon, Butter, and
    Caper Sauce, 216
Panna Cotta (Italian Custard),
    260
Parisian Hot Chocolate, 261
Parmesan:
    and Arugula Salad, 174
    Asparagus with Butter and,
      195
    Bowls with Caesar Salad,
      172
    Chips, 170
    Creamy Sauce, 135
    Croutons, 171
    Crusts, Baby Lamb Chops
      with Sweet Tomato Sauce
      and, 234–35
    Eggplant, 207
    Fennel with Butter and,
      197
    Spinach Frittata, 138
Parsley and Red Bean Salad,
    179
Pastas:
    Hearty Mushroom Lasagna,
      186
    whole-grain, 98, 123
    Whole-Grain, Primavera,
      187
Peanut butter, 121
Peas, Gingered Snap, 199
Peppered Filet of Beef with
    Bourbon Sauce, 244
Pepper(s):
    Red, Eggs Baked in Toma-
      toes and, 136
    Roasted, 165
    Roasted Sweet Red, Soup
      with Crème Fraiche and
      Crispy Sage Leaves,
      164–65

Pesto:
    Artichoke, 154
    Basil, 155
    Bubbling, Portobello Mush-
      rooms with, 200
    Fondue with Sausages, 218
    Sun-Dried Tomato, 156
Pickles, 121
Pork:
    Baby Back Ribs, 230
    Chops with Creamy Shallot
      Sauce, 228
    Rosemary Roast Loin of,
      229
Portion control, 100–101, 122
Portobello Mushrooms with
    Bubbling Pesto, 200
Poultry, 99, 217–25
    Deep-Fried Turkey with
      Fried Onions and Herbs,
      220
    see also Chicken
Pregnant women, 43, 45
Premarin, xviii
Prime Rib au Jus with Garlic
    Crust, 246–47
Pro/Fats, 10, 27, 76–77,
      105–7, 267–68, 270
Progesterone, xviii, 56
Protein Power, 15, 17
Proteins:
    as building blocks, 36, 39
    burning off, 8
    in commercial diet plans, 3
    and food combining, 46
    in Pro/Fats group, 76–77
    separation from carbohy-
      drates, 1
Pumpernickel bagels, 122

Quick Chicken Broth, 161

Raspberry Soufflé, 253
Red Bean and Parsley Salad,
    179

Red Hot Singing Scallops, 211
Red Wine Butter Sauce, 157
Red Wine Vinaigrette, 153
Reference guide, 267–70
Restaurants, 95–96, 118
Ribs, Baby Back Pork, 230
Rich Mocha Coolers, 143
Ricotta and Spinach Filling,
    Egg Crêpes with, 133
Roasted Peppers, 165
Roasted Sweet Red Pepper
    Soup with Crème Fraiche
    and Crispy Sage Leaves,
    164–65
Roasted Turkey Gravy, 158
Root Beer Float, 255
Rosemary-Infused Savory
    Custard with Tomato
    Mushroom Sauce,
    192–93
Rosemary Roast Loin of Pork,
    229
Rye Bread, 183

Sage Leaves, Fried, 165
Salad dressings, 117
    Caesar, 173
    Green Goddess, 149
    Lemon Tarragon Vinai-
      grette, 152
    Red Wine Vinaigrette, 153
    see also specific salads
Salads, 169–80
    à la Niçoise, 177
    Arugula and Parmesan, 174
    Caesar, 173
    Hearts of Palm and Green
      Bean, 176
    Israeli, 175
    Red Bean and Parsley, 179
    Southern Country Fried
      Chicken, 178
    Tabbouleh, 185
    White Bean, with Sage and
      Thyme, 180

Salsa, Tarragon, 232
Salsa de Perez, 151
Sauces:
    Balsamic Syrup, 224
    Bourbon, 244
    Creamy Parmesan, 135
    Creamy Shallot, 228
    Lemon, Butter, and Caper, 216
    Meat, 238
    Mozzarella Marinara, 130
    Red Wine Butter, 157
    Roasted Turkey Gravy, 158
    Salsa de Perez, 151
    Sweet Tomato, 235
    Tarragon Salsa, 232
    Tomato Mushroom, 193
Sausages:
    Jalapeño Chili, 240–41
    Pesto Fondue with, 218
Sautéed Spinach with Garlic, Lemon, and Oil, 201
Scallops, Red Hot Singing, 211
Schwarzbein, Diana, 2, 13, 22, 28–29, 32, 42, 56–59
Seafood:
    fresh, 99
    see also Fish and shellfish
Serotonin, 76
Shallot Sauce, Creamy, 228
Shellfish, *see* Fish and shellfish
Shrimp:
    Grilled Ginger, on Skewers, 213
    Pan-Fried Garlic Lemon, with Zucchini Pesto Noodles and Arugula, 214
Side dishes, 189–207
    Asparagus with Butter and Parmesan, 195
    Black Bean Vegetable Chili, 204–5
    Caramelized Fennel, 196
    Chinese Long Beans, 198

    Eggplant Parmesan, 207
    Fennel with Butter and Parmesan Cheese, 197
    Gingered Snap Peas, 199
    Green Chili Celery Root Puree, 190
    Grilled Artichokes, 194
    Grilled Vegetable Antipasto, 191
    Middle Eastern Vegetable Stew, 206
    Portobello Mushrooms with Bubbling Pesto, 200
    Rosemary-Infused Savory Custard with Tomato Mushroom Sauce, 192–93
    Sautéed Spinach with Garlic, Lemon, and Oil, 201
    Spicy Broccoli, 202
    Zucchini Noodles, 203
Simple carbohydrates, 23
Snacks, 117
Sole, Pan-Fried Petrale, with Lemon, Butter, and Caper Sauce, 216
Somersize Zucchini Muffins, 128
Somersizing:
    basic tenets of, 18
    for children, 60–67
    commitment to, 70
    compared to other eating plans, 18–19
    dining out with, 95–96
    and energy levels, 48
    food categories in, 10–11, 75
    food combining in, 46–52
    foods eliminated in, 72, 74–75
    foods separated in, 75–81
    idea of, 1
    Level One, 11–13, 25, 52, 83–102
    Level Two, 103–14

    name of, 2
    questions about, 115–23
    seven easy steps to, 11
    tips, 95–96
    unique qualities of, 3
    for vegetarians, 78
    as a way of life, 14
    why people like or don't like it, 18–19
Somersizing success stories:
    access/address, 113–14
    Alexander, Sandy and Peter, 16–17
    Bertrand, Cecile, 113
    Burcham, Angie, 119
    Clancy, Barbara, 47
    Daley, Karen, 44
    DeRose, Paula, 102
    Fossitt, Lois S., 62
    Gamsky, Verna, 33
    Hetherington, Sue, 69
    Layton, Roberta, 12
    Lewandowski, Cheryl, 80
    Love, Jody, 71
    Lutonsky, Rebecca-Rose, 28
    Scott, Lisa, 51
    Tworney, Wendy, 38
    Zigler, John, 9
SomerSweet, 25, 73–74, 92–93, 108–9
Soufflé, Raspberry, 253
Soups, 159–67
    Beef Stew, 242
    Chicken Meatball Asparagus, 163
    Cream of Green Chili, 160
    Middle Eastern Vegetable Stew, 206
    Quick Chicken Broth, 161
    Roasted Sweet Red Pepper, with Crème Fraiche and Crispy Sage Leaves, 164–65
    Stracciatella, 166
    Watercress Mushroom, 167

Southern Country Fried
     Chicken Salad, 178
Soy products, 122
Spicy Broccoli, 202
Spinach:
   Dip, 148
   Parmesan Frittata, 138
   and Ricotta Filling, Egg
        Crêpes with, 133
   Sautéed, with Garlic,
        Lemon, and Oil, 201
Starches:
   and blood sugar, 48
   as carbohydrates, 21
   elimination of, 74–75, 270
   stored as fat, 47
Steak Florentine, 247
Stevia, 73
Stews:
   Beef, 242
   Middle Eastern Vegetable,
        206
Stir-Fry, Beef, 243
Stracciatella Soup, 166
Sugar:
   blood, 21, 22, 23, 24, 48
   as carbohydrate, 21
   children and, 60, 61
   and cholesterol, 2
   as comfort food, 20
   elimination of, 46, 72, 270
   as enemy, 2, 3, 4, 19, 54
   and heart disease, 2
   nature of, 23–25
   research on, 13
   stored as fat, 37, 39, 47
   the truth about, 20–25
Sugar Busters, 18
Sugar-free foods, 121
Sugarless Fudgysicles, 252
"Sugar low," 24
"Sugar rush" or "sugar high,"
     23

Sun-Dried Tomato Pesto, 156
Suppression therapy, xix
Survival instinct, 8–10
Sweet Tomato Sauce, 235
Swiss Cheese Fondue, 236

*T*abbouleh, 185
Tamoxifen, 123
Tarragon Lemon Vinaigrette,
     152
Tarragon Salsa, 232
Tea, Fresh Mint, 142
Testosterone, 56
Tofu, 116
Tomato(es):
   Eggs Baked in Red Peppers
        and, 136
   Mushroom Sauce, 193
   Sun-Dried, Pesto, 156
   Sweet Sauce, 235
Tracking, xix
Trans fats, 29–30
Triterpene glycosides, 73
Truffles, Chocolate, 263
Turkey, Deep-Fried, with
        Fried Onions and Herbs,
        220
Turkey Gravy, Roasted, 158
Type II diabetes, 23, 33,
     265–66

*V*anilla Bean Ice Cream, 250
Vegetable Antipasto, Grilled,
     191
Vegetable Black Bean Chili,
     204–5
Vegetable Stew, Middle East-
     ern, 206
Vegetarians, 78
Veggie burgers, 117

Veggies, 10, 77, 78, 99, 269,
     270; *see also* Side dishes
Vinaigrettes:
   Lemon Tarragon, 152
   Red Wine, 153
Vinegar, 99
Vitamins, 34, 77

*W*ater, 117–18
Watercress Mushroom Soup,
     167
Water weight, use of term, 8
Weight gain:
   causes of, 19, 57–58
   lifestyle and, 41–42
Weight loss:
   for children, 60
   cutting calories for, 7–8
   in Level One, 11–13, 25, 52
White Bean Salad with Sage
     and Thyme, 180
Whole-grain breads, 97–98,
     116
Whole-Grain Pasta Primavera,
     187
Whole Wheat Bread, 182
Wine, 110
   Red, Butter Sauce, 157
   Red, Vinaigrette, 153

*Y*ogurt, 119–20

*Z*one, The, 17–18
Zucchini:
   Noodles, 203
   Pesto Noodles, Pan-Fried
        Garlic Lemon Shrimp
        with Arugula and, 214
   Somersize Muffins, 128

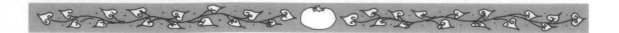

About the Author

SUZANNE SOMERS is the author of seven books, including the New York Times bestsellers *Keeping Secrets; Eat Great, Lose Weight;* and *Get Skinny on Fabulous Food.* The former star of the hit television programs *Three's Company* and *Step by Step,* Suzanne Somers is also responsible for the wildly successful ThighMaster fitness products and her own line of jewelry on the Home Shopping Network.

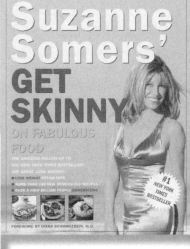
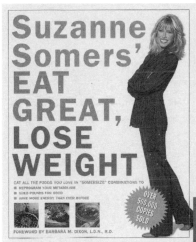
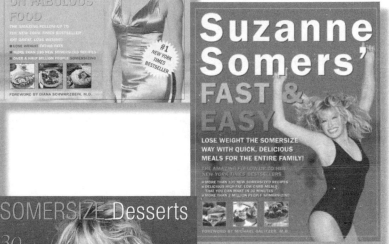

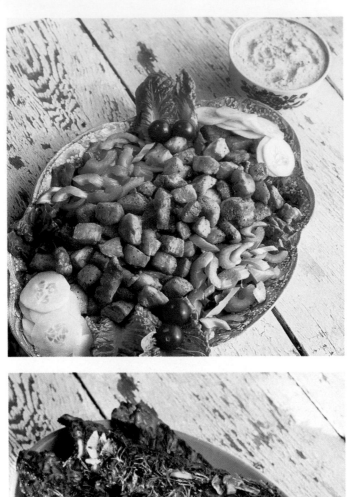

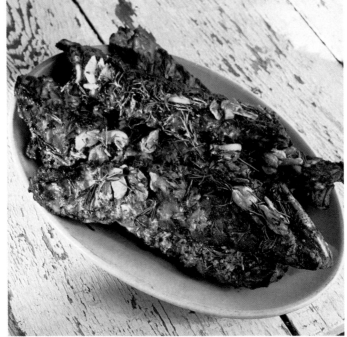

PREVIOUS PAGES: Enjoying a lovely Somersized picnic with my girls.

TOP: Southern Country Fried Chicken Salad

BOTTOM: Baby Back Pork Ribs

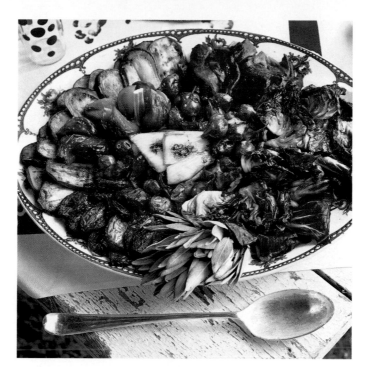

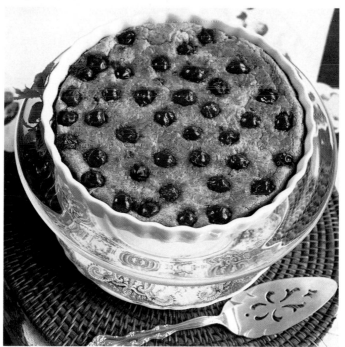

TOP: Grilled Vegetable Antipasto
BOTTOM: Cherry Claflouti

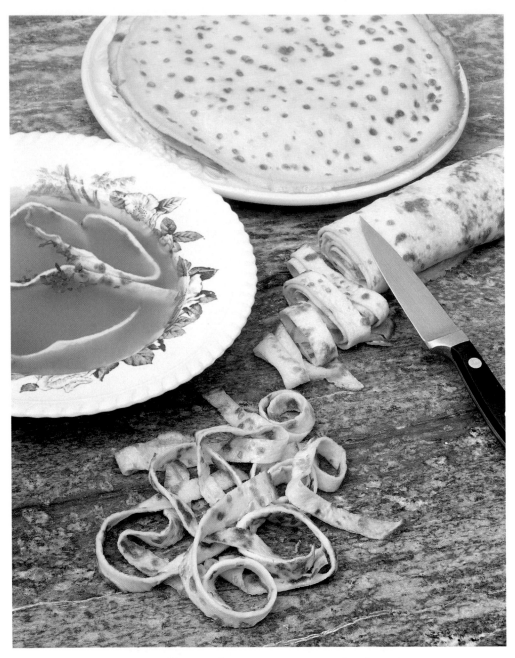

Making egg noodles is a breeze—you can make them from my
Egg Crêpes recipe. And they taste great in soup.

reduced smoking and drinking. The control group only had a checkup once a year. At the end of the five-year study, those who had reduced their smoking, drinking, and cholesterol intake had decreased the rate of heart disease and death by 47 percent over those who did not.

The results were certainly dramatic and made a serious impression on the medical community. These results, however, were grossly misinterpreted. The intervention group's lower cholesterol levels were attributed solely to eating less cholesterol (meat, eggs, butter, etc.) and so the "fat-free" movement began. But what the study didn't document was the *insulin* levels in the intervention group as opposed to the control group's. The intervention group's decreased consumption of sugar, alcohol, and smoking was not even considered a contributing effect in lowering cholesterol levels! And we know anything that lowers your insulin levels will create multiple benefits including weight loss, lower cholesterol levels, and decreased risk of heart disease. What the intervention group *actually* showed was that decreasing smoking cigarettes, drinking less alcohol, and eating less sugar lowers insulin levels. And these lower insulin levels decreased cholesterol.

Because of this study, and the misinterpreted results, we've all been taught for the last two decades that eating less cholesterol will help lower cholesterol levels. One study has changed the opinion about what connotes "healthy" eating. And remember, there are *no* long-term studies proving the negative effects of fat. All the hoopla in the fat-free movement is based on short-term

studies. Meanwhile, as a society we've replaced dinners revolving around some kind of protein with meals predominantly made up of carbohydrates. To be more "healthy" we've replaced steak dinners with pasta dinners and pork chops with fried rice. Everything has become low-fat, but even though we've cut our fat intake in the last two decades, we've gained weight, increased our cholesterol, and the incidence of cancer. The low-fat movement is not working! Carbohydrates are fuel for energy, but think about your car . . . it needs gas for fuel, but imagine how your engine would falter if you never gave it any oil! Your body needs "oil" too, which is why you must include fats and protein in your diet—to keep your engine running smoothly.

Question #8: Is Somersizing safe for pregnant or nursing women?

Pregnancy is a very special time in a woman's life. Your body is housing and building another life and you must make sure to provide your baby with all the necessary nutrients. Actually, if you do not eat a proper diet, your baby will take the nutrients it needs from your body. It will break down your muscles and bones if you are not eating enough protein and calcium. So if you are eating a poor diet, your baby may still be fine, but *your* body will greatly suffer!

Most doctors recommend that pregnant women eat at least 100 grams of protein per day. Proteins are the building blocks for the human body—yours and your baby's. You also need to make sure to get plenty of calcium. Somersizing on Level Two (the main-

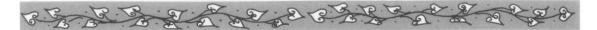

Dear Suzanne:

Like so many others, Somersizing has changed my life. I never was extremely overweight, but like everyone else, have struggled to stay slim and lose those last 10 pounds by starving myself and exercising way too much. This continued all through college and until after the birth of my second child. She was four months old, and there I sat, 25 pounds overweight and starving myself again. I was miserable! Then I saw you on TV and you were talking about how you could eat all this great food and still lose weight. Since I had always admired you, and because I was starving, I decided to get your book that afternoon. Once I started reading, I couldn't put it down.

The very next day I started Somersizing, and within less than three months I lost every last one of those 25 pounds. It was effortless. I ate until I was full at every meal and even had two snacks a day. I was in heaven! People can't believe I eat the way I do. When I became pregnant for the third time, I decided to stick with it during the pregnancy. My doctor thought that it was a very balanced way of eating and was also glad that it did not contain any chemicals and processed foods. I gained only 21 pounds. Shortly after having my daughter, I was showing her off wearing my jeans. What a great feeling!

I began an exercise program with my friend Michele, and now I work out with her class for one hour, four days a week, instead of two hours a day, seven days a week like I did before. It has now been over three and a half years since I bought your book, and I am currently at a healthy weight of 122 pounds. I enjoy my food instead of obsessing over it. I will eat this way for life.

Thank you, Suzanne.

Sincerely,
Karen Daley

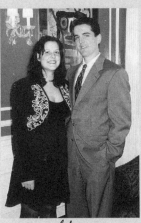

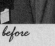

before

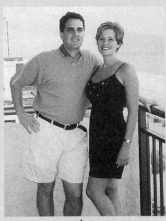

after

tenance portion of the program) is perfect for pregnant women! Check with your doctor. I'm sure he/she will endorse Somersizing. You eat food rich in protein, real fats, and calcium—chicken, beef, fish, turkey, and more. Cheese, milk, yogurt, cottage cheese, and more. And unlike other high-protein programs, we include whole-grain carbohydrates, vegetables low in starch, and fresh fruit. The only things eliminated from the program are sugar and foods high in starch. These foods are empty calories that do not provide you or your baby any type of nutrition.

Many pregnant women worry about gaining weight. If you eat the Somersize way, you will gain only the weight your baby needs. If you use pregnancy as an excuse to eat anything you want, you will gain weight that will be difficult to take off. Whether you're pregnant or not, filling up on sugar and starches, like potatoes, white bread, and sugar, will lead to weight gain. Don't eat extra junk, thinking it doesn't matter if you gain weight because you're fat from your pregnancy anyway. The average 25–35 pounds you will gain will come off quickly if you eat healthy foods while you are pregnant.

As for nursing women, Somersizing on Level One is the perfect solution to losing weight while eating all the foods you need to make milk for your baby. Again, while you are nursing you need to make sure you are getting enough protein, fat, and calcium. If you are not eating enough of these foods, your body will break down your muscles and bones to create the milk your baby needs. And if you cut back your calories in an attempt to lose the weight from your pregnancy, you put your milk supply at risk. Many women lose their milk from cutting their calories and fat while nursing. When you Somersize, you give your body the protein, real fat, and calcium it needs to create milk for your baby, and you melt away your pregnancy pounds at the same time. And because you are eating plenty of food, you are increasing your metabolism, building lean muscle mass, and supplying your baby with the most nutritious food you can give him or her.

SIX

Food Combining: Fact or Fad?

Somersizing has helped over two million people lose weight and gain vital energy while they heal their systems from years of bad food and lifestyle choices. But even after losing 10, 20, 30 pounds or more, many people still don't understand how a program with this much food and this much flavor can help you lose weight and feel healthier.

The theory behind food combining is that proteins and carbohydrates digest at different rates of speed. Proteins require an acid environment to be digested and carbohydrates require a base environment. When eaten togther the enzymes cancel each other out, creating a halt in the digestion process. Many food-combining advocates support this theory; however, there are challengers who argue that food combining is not based on scientific facts.

Here's what I know: food combining works. Over two million of you have proven that to me and, frankly, that's all the proof I need! *Why* does it work? Although I am not a doctor or a nutritionist, I will try to explain how Somersizing works in the layman's terms I have come to understand. These are the facts that are scientifically proven when it comes to Somersizing:

When you eliminate sugar, white flour, and other Funky Foods, you force your body to burn off your fat reserves and use them as an energy source. That's how you melt the fat away!

Eliminating sugar and foods high in starch, like potatoes and white rice, is the essential reason why we lose weight on the Somersize system. Carbohydrates are one of the body's main sources of energy. Carbs are the fuel that keeps us going. But, as we've learned, it is important to be eating the *right kind* of carbohydrates. Whole grains, fruits, and vegetables low in starch are excellent sources of carbohydrates that give us energy and provide necessary fiber for proper elimination. But some carbohydrates, like sugar and foods very high in starch, are loaded with more energy than our bodies can use at a given time. This excess energy that isn't burned off will be stored as fat for later use. (Of course, your activity level determines that quotient.)

I cannot stress enough how crucial it is to understand that *sugar is more fattening than fat.* Even though sugars and starches are "fat free," they have a tendency to turn right to fat. Think of a baked potato as one gigantic sugar cube and imagine the amount of excess energy you are giving your body! At first I grieved the loss of potatoes in my diet. As a child I practically lived on potatoes and salad. My grandfather was a butcher and he would bring my mother the meat and fish they could no longer sell because it was beginning to turn. My mother would soak it in vinegar to remove the odor, but as far as I was concerned it smelled and tasted rancid. I picked around the stinky meat or fish and lived on the side dishes, potatoes and salad.

As a child I had no problem metabolizing the sugar from the potato, but when I hit my forties I started gaining weight. When I think not only about the potatoes, but about the *kind* of carbs and the *amount* of carbs I used to eat, I understand why I was gaining weight: toast or cereal in the morning, a sandwich for lunch, and pasta or meat

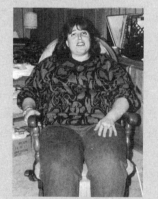

Hello Suzanne!

I just had to let you know how great your eating plan is. I had a stroke 13 years ago when I was 29 years old. While I was in hospital (for eight weeks), my family used to bring me "goodies," all sorts of things like donuts, cakes, candies, chocolate bars, etc. I know they felt sorry for me as I was a young woman in a situation where everyone around me was elderly. At the time, not knowing basically which way was up, I gorged myself on all the food. I have tried time and time again to lose the weight to no avail. I have since lost 35 pounds on your eating plan and still have a ways to go, but I LOVE IT! It is so easy—and I find that I am not craving foods. Only one thing, though—I do miss white bread! Anyways, that is what I wanted you to know—I can see success for the first time in years.

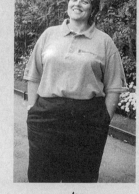

before

after

Sincerely,
Barbara Clancy

with potatoes for dinner adds up to way more energy than I needed to get through the day with my slower forty-year-old metabolism. All that extra sugar had no place to be stored in my cells, so it was converted to fat and not burned off.

Sugar and foods high in starch can also put your blood sugar levels on a roller coaster, which keeps you hungry and tired. When you eat sugar or starch, your blood sugar increases and you feel great. That's when your metabolism says, "Hey, this sugar rush is fun. I've got all sorts of energy!" But before the blood sugar is back to normal it usually dips *below* its starting point. It is during this "sugar low" that your metabolism will say, "Whoa, what happened to all the fun? I feel awful; tired, listless, or am I hungry? Hey, up there, how about a little pick-me-up?" That's often when we decide to reach for more sugar or caffeine to pick up our energy level. Well, watch the cycle repeat itself . . . we have a few cookies and our blood sugar increases. At first we feel good, then our blood sugar decreases to below its starting point and we feel tired and hungry. Once again, we reach for something sweet or caffeinated to keep our energy level up. In goes the candy bar, up goes the blood sugar, down goes the blood sugar, and so on and so on and so on. Sugars and certain starches are empty foods that cause highs and lows in our energy level, which can cause us to eat way more than our actual appetites require. Don't be tricked by your metabolism. Once you start bingeing on sugar or carbohydrates, your body will crave more and more of these empty foods. You must know better and give your body what it is actually craving—proteins, real fats, and vegetables that will give your body everything it needs to thrive.

When you Somersize, your energy level remains constant. You can eat as much as you want, but you will not overeat because you are giving your body good nutritious foods that satisfy your appetite. It is not calories that lead to weight gain—it's imbalanced hormones. That is why you may eat until you are full . . . period.

Here's what I might eat in a typical day: Fried eggs with sautéed spinach and onions and crisp bacon. Midmorning I might snack on a piece of cheese. For lunch, a hearty salad with grilled chicken and full fat salad dressing. Maybe a piece of fruit in the afternoon as a snack. And for dinner? Chicken, meat or fish with a lovely sauce, plenty of fresh sautéed, steamed, or grilled vegetables, and a green salad with full fat dressing of my choice. And guess what? Without sugar and highly starchy foods to turn to for quick energy sources, our bodies have to look elsewhere to provide us with vital energy . . . and guess where they look first? Our fat reserves! Our fat reserves become our bodies' vital energy source. That layer of fat starts melting away while we are infused with energy—all the while eating delicious, nutritious foods loaded with flavor.

I hope that after reading this far, you have come to realize that fat is not your enemy. Eating real foods in the proper combinations will lead to weight loss and greater health. Despite the compelling evidence I've shared with you about this, it is sometimes hard for people to understand that it is always better to eat real food, including fat, instead of the fat-free alternative. In *Get Skinny on Fabulous Food,* I came up with a great way to show readers why they should steer clear of fat-free products by sharing the ingredient lists of full-fat and fat-free products. Below, you can see the different lists.

Notice how much farther away we get from real food as we take the fat out of mayonnaise. The eggs and oil get replaced with sugar and starches. By the time you get to the fat-free Miracle Whip, you can hardly pronounce a single ingredient! Imagine what's happening to your body by ingesting a lifetime of chemicals and preservatives. How can anyone think that picking the fat-free product is the healthy option? How? Because we've been trained to look at only fat grams and calories. Yes, the low-fat and no-fat

products are lower in fat and calories, but fat causes no insulin response and therefore will not be converted to fat. The sugars and starches, however, cause a rise in blood sugar, which triggers an insulin response, which can cause fat-free mayonnaise to be stored as fat.

There is a fascinating ongoing ten-year study called the Nurses Health Study, which is tracking the diets and heart disease of 76,000 women. One of the major differences between those who stayed healthy and those who did not was the amount of oil-based salad dressings they ate. Those who stayed healthy included essential fats in their diet, predominantly by eating mayonnaise, creamy salad dressing, and oil-and-vinegar dressings five or more times a week. Those who developed heart disease or died ate these foods

MAYONNAISE:

My Homemade Mayonnaise (from *Eat Great, Lose Weight*)

Vegetable oil, eggs, vinegar, lemon juice, salt, white pepper, tabasco, Worcestershire
Calories per tablespoon: 100
Fat grams: 11 g

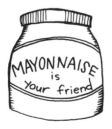

Best Foods Mayonnaise

Soybean oil, eggs, vinegar, water, salt, lemon juice, natural flavors, calcium disodium EDTA used to protect quality
Calories per tablespoon: 100
Fat grams: 11 g

Best Foods Low-Fat Mayonnaise Dressing

Water, corn syrup, soybean oil, modified food starch, egg whites, vinegar, salt, maltodextrin, gums (cellulose gel and gum), xanthan, carrageenan, natural flavors, color added, mustard flour, sodium benzoate, calcium disodium EDTA used to protect quality
Calories per tablespoon: 25
Fat grams: 1 g

Kraft Miracle Whip Nonfat Dressing

Water, sugar, natural and artificial flavor (contains egg*), modified food starch, vinegar, contains less than 2% of cellulose gel, salt, citric acid, xanthan gum, dried cream*, artificial color, lactic acid, with potassium sorbate and calcium disodium EDTA as preservatives, yellow 6, phylloquinone (vitamin K1), blue 1

*trivial source of fat and cholesterol

Calories per tablespoon: 15
Fat grams: 0 g

only rarely. Please! Eat full-fat products in their natural state. Your taste buds, your thighs, and your heart will thank you.

Let's look at the ice cream examples I've listed below.

Again, look at the sugars, starches, and chemicals that take the place of real food when you extract the fat from ice cream. It's easy to think you're making a healthier choice by picking the fat-free item if you look only at the calories and fat. I wish these products had an insulin meter on the labels so we could see the effect on our blood sugar and the subsequent insulin levels. One reading that helps give some insight is the carbohydrate count. The real ice cream has 15 grams of carbohydrate per serving, while the fat-free product has 23 grams. The higher carbohydrate count means more insulin and all the negativity that comes with it. Plus, many people eat larger portions of fat-free products because they think there is no harm in eating something that is fat free. If you're going to eat ice cream make my incredible sugarless Vanilla Bean ice cream. It's made with SomerSweet so it won't cause any insulin response (read more about SomerSweet on page 73). Or, in Level Two, eat a moderate amount of full fat ice cream, like Breyer's, after a Pro/Fats meal for the least amount of imbalance.

Now let's analyze some breakfast meals, listed below, to see the effect of sugars and fats.

ICE CREAM:

Breyer's Natural Vanilla

milk, cream, sugar, natural vanilla flavor
Calories per 1/2 cup: 150
Fat grams: 9 g
Carbohydrates: 15 g

Dreyer's Fat Free Ice Cream

skim milk, sugar, corn syrup, modified food starch, natural and artificial flavor, cellulose gel, cellulose gum, mono and diglycerides, tara gum, carrageenan, dextrose, vitamin A, palmitate, annatto color
Calories per 1/2 cup: 100
Fat grams: 0 g
Carbohydrates: 23 g

BREAKFAST MEALS:

Two eggs fried in butter (1 tablespoon) Three pork sausage links One sliced tomato

Calories: 425
Fat grams: 35 g
Carbohydrates: 1.5 g

Awrey's Raisin Bran Muffin

Calories: 320
Fat grams: 12 g
Carbohydrates: 50 g

Healthy Choice Low-Fat Apple Spice Muffin:

Calories: 190
Fat grams: 4 g
Carbohydrates: 40 g

Hungry Jack Buttermilk Pancakes (3) with butter (1 tablespoon) and maple syrup (3 tablespoons):

Calories: 490
Fat grams: 15 g
Carbohydrates: 90

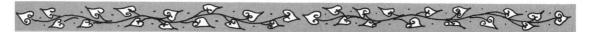

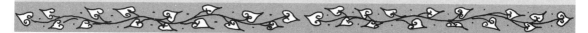

If you were to place these breakfast options side by side and ask someone to rate them from the most healthful to the least healthful, they would probably rate either of the muffins as the most healthful, then the pancakes, leaving the fried eggs and sausage as the least healthful. But look at the carbohydrate content in the muffins: the apple spice muffin has 40, and the raisin bran muffin has a whopping 50 grams of carbohydrate. For many of us, that's more than we need for an entire day! Don't be fooled, folks. These muffins are just an excuse to eat cake in the morning. Just because they contain apples, or bran, or may be low-fat doesn't mean they are healthy options. They are also loaded with sugar and, commonly, white flour, which will send the insulin soaring. (Try my Somersize Zucchini Muffins!) Pancakes (made from white flour) with butter and maple syrup, are, not surprisingly, loaded with bad carbohydrates (90 grams!). If you're going to eat pancakes, you're much

better off making pancakes from buckwheat or whole wheat flour and topping them with yogurt and raspberry sauce. (Or try my Oatmeal Pancake recipe in *Get Skinny on Fabulous Food*.) Then we have the fried eggs and sausage, a meal that has only trace amounts of carbohydrates. That means there is no insulin response, and if there is no presence of insulin, then food cannot be stored as fat. I know it's hard to believe, but I didn't make this stuff up. It's based on medical research. And as far as cholesterol is concerned, I covered the real culprit for clogged arteries—raised insulin levels—at length in the previous chapter.

For those carbohydrate addicts who say, "I can't give up my pastries and bagels in the morning!" or "I just have to eat something sweet in the middle of the afternoon!" these cravings will pass. At first you may feel as though you are making substantial sacrifices by not eating the pasta, pizza, potatoes, cookies, cakes, and candy to which your body may be accustomed. As your system unloads the built-up sugar from your cells, your cravings for these types of sugar and carbohydrates will diminish. Some people *ease* their way into the program by weaning away from these foods for the first week or two, until they cut them out completely and then diligently begin Level One on the third week or so. This way they are not asking their bodies to go "cold turkey" away from the sweets and bad carbohydrates that keep them overweight and unhealthy. Others decide to just go for it and begin this new lifestyle full force from day one. I recommend you try the latter.

Either way, I will tell you there is no way to lose weight magically. Nothing is totally free. In fact, I was on a set recently, explaining the program to my friend Matt, who told me he wanted to try it. Another friend (who is skinny as a rail) was discouraging Matt, saying, "You don't want to do that. You can't eat any bread. You can't eat pasta. No cake after lunch!" He's right. Sure, if you compare Somersizing to *no* diet at all, it feels restrictive, but compared to a low-calorie/low-fat diet, Somersizing is a plea-

sure. You do have to give up something, but the benefits of the Somersize system far outweigh the restrictions. So you can't eat sugar and white bread . . . but look at what you can eat! Butter, eggs, cream, sour cream, olive oil, cheese, whole grains, fresh vegetables, fruit, a huge variety of meats, and delicious sauces! That's right . . . when I want butter or cream or eggs or cheese, I eat it. Hardly a sacrifice at all to lose all the weight you want, gain vital energy, and keep you at your metabolic prime in order to stave off disease. Thankfully, Matt ignored the doubter and started to Somersize. I am proud to report he lost eighteen pounds in the first month and has kept all the weight off for a year!

As soon as Matt reached his goal weight he began Level Two and started enjoying some sugars and starches in moderation. Soon you'll be at your goal weight, too, incorporating some sugars and starches without gaining the weight back. Because come on, every now and then you just have to have a little something sweet. Just make sure it's really worth it.

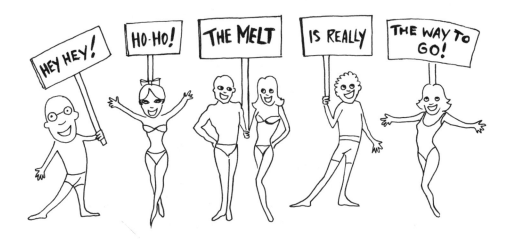

Change the Way You Think, Forever, About Dieting and Eating

SEVEN

Hormonal Balance

When we talk about hormonal imbalance, many people immediately think of menopause (or as I refer to it, "men-on-pause"). But if you think hormonal imbalance is reserved only for middle-aged women, think again. You can be hormonally out of whack at any age. It affects men, women, even children. And the symptoms of imbalanced hormones can be devastating.

Remember feeling berserk when you were a teenager? That's because your hormones were in a state of flux. For many, that's when we started gaining weight and experiencing the embarrassment of acne. Consider the mood swings many of us women experience during our monthly cycle. To this day, there is one day a month when I just cannot stand my husband. I go from being madly in love with him one day to not being able to think of a single reason why I married him! Or think about pregnant women with that glowing skin. That

glow doesn't come in a bottle—it's from hormones. Why does pregnancy change some women's hair from curly to straight? Why do some go gray? Why do women lose their sex drive just after giving birth? Why do some experience postpartem depression?

Complexion? Hormones. Depression? Hormones. Elation? Hormones. Sex drive? Hormones. The list goes on and on. The bottom line is that hormones rule our lives. Excess weight gain is also a hormonal problem. Think about the overweight child in school. Everyone always assumes that overweight kids are just lazy and have no willpower. Often, nothing could be further from the truth. Many people, including children, have a hard time metabolizing sugar. That overweight kid may eat no differently than the stick figure next to him, but if he has difficulty metabolizing sugar, he may begin a lifelong battle with obesity and the humiliation that accompanies it. We feed our children a diet of sugar. Many of us are not aware of hidden sugars in cereal, milk, peanut butter, jelly, white bread, chips, bananas, hot dogs, white pasta, and apple juice. These are all forms of sugar and many children survive on little else, thus throwing their hormones out of balance, leading to possible weight gain, irritability, and greater susceptibility to disease. I will discuss more about how vital it is to make sure our children eat right in Chapter 8. It's not just children, though, who are hormonally sensitive to what they eat. People at every age can experience elevated insulin levels from eating sugar, which can lead to weight gain. When we are "insulin resistant," weight gain is far more likely. This condition can develop in childhood, or one can slowly accumulate insulin resistance as the years go by. As I said, the most telling way to know if your insulin levels are elevated is to stand naked in front of the mirror. If you are thick around the middle, your insulin levels are too high. This means that your cells, which store the sugars you ingest, are *loaded*. From that moment on, *any* sugars you ingest, in any form, are going to be stored as fat.

Since sugar raises insulin levels, and insulin is the fat-storing hormone, it becomes clear why so many of us have been on a hormonal merry-go-round for most of our lives. If our insulin levels are raised, our entire hormonal system can be thrown out of balance. That imbalance can cause weight gain, and risk of disease and early death. That's the bad news. The good news is that elevated insulin levels are infinitely curable! Somersizing is designed to change your eat-

ing habits, cure your insulin resistance, and get you off the carousel.

MENOPAUSE, OR "MEN-ON-PAUSE"

But what if you are Somersizing correctly and exercising but still gaining weight? How can this happen if you are eating properly and thus balancing your hormones? Although Somersizing can balance some of your hormones, it cannot solve all hormonal imbalances, particularly as women get older. Before middle age, Somersizing may be enough to keep your hormones in check. But as women approach middle age, we begin to lose the sex hormones: estrogen, progesterone, and testosterone. If you are taking care of yourself, eliminating stress as best you can, exercising, eating properly, not drinking caffeine, not taking drugs (prescription, over-the-counter, or recreational), and you find that you are gaining weight anyway, you may be a candidate for hormone replacement.

Here are the symptoms I experienced. Without warning, I suddenly had no interest in sex. None. In addition, I was Somersizing with my usual cheating, but now I found I was getting a little thick around my waistline. I stopped all cheating, but the weight wasn't going away; in fact I seemed to be putting on a little more weight. I panicked, because Somersizing had been working perfectly for me for ten years. I couldn't figure out what I was doing wrong. I felt bewildered because there is very little information available for those of us entering this new passage. Our mothers must have pretended it was not happening, because I can't ever remember my mother talking about menopause or complaining about the various symptoms, including decreased sex drive. I had no idea that loss of libido is due to decreased estrogen levels and is a symptom that can be treated, not an irreversible condition.

Rest assured, I have figured out this tricky new stage and am enjoying this phase of my life immensely, although it took some sleuthing. In passing along what I have learned researching menopause, I would like to stress the importance of checking with your own doctor before changing the way you have been approaching your health. I have no way of knowing your particular health risks, and it is necessary for you to evaluate changes with your own particular health history in mind.

I feel strongly that it is important to be proactive about your health. As a general rule, I have found that the medical community gets comfortable with the information taught in medical school (no matter how long ago it may have been), and more often than not does not keep up with the latest studies. I still cannot believe how little information there is out there about a natural phase of life that will affect *every woman* fortunate enough to live to middle age. When I first started experiencing the symptoms of menopause, one doctor told me to go to the health food store and buy black Cohosh and a lot of other useless herbs and supplements. (I am very pro vitamins and herbs, but believe me, they provide very little relief when you're suffering from decreased estrogen.) Another told me it was

"just a phase to be endured; after all, in days of old, we women would have died off after our childbearing years, so you should appreciate the fact you are living longer than your predecessors, even if it is a little uncomfortable." A little uncomfortable! I'd like to see him sail through insomnia, unbelievable fatigue, weight gain, hot flashes, short-term memory loss, unexplained rashes, vaginal dryness, bitchiness, and the feeling that everyone has the heat turned up full blast in every office building, home, and restaurant in America! No wonder menopausal women have been the butt of jokes for ages. It's hard to find the humor when you haven't had a good night's sleep in weeks.

In my case, life was good, and then all of a sudden I felt like I was living in someone else's body. The first devastating symptom, as I mentioned, was no interest in sex (thus "men-on-pause"). It made me feel confused and a bit sad, like I was losing an old friend. I figured it was because I was working long hours and not giving myself enough down time. I vowed to take time off. Then came the hot flashes, night sweats, and an inability to remember even the simplest phone numbers. I started to feel a panic inside, like I was losing my mind or something.

My gynecologist told me it was nothing to worry about, that I was "of age" and that it was time to think about hormone replacement therapy. "There's Premarin, Provera, or methyltestosterone," she told me. "They are synthetic hormones that take all the guesswork out of it. Just slap that estrogen patch on your arm and all your symptoms will disappear." I was concerned about synthetic hormones, because I had read that they simply remove the symptoms, but do nothing to actually replace lost hormones. When I asked my doctor about this, she replied, "It's the symptoms that are bothering you. These pills will take care of that." I realized that although my doctor knew her stuff about delivering babies, dealing with the occasional yeast infection, and my yearly Pap smear, she was uninformed about hormone replacement.

I decided to try another doctor. All the while I was having trouble sleeping, felt exhausted during the day, couldn't hold a thought, didn't want sex, and was constantly on the verge of tears. I was becoming desperate. The next doctor came highly recommended, and we began the process again. "I don't want to take synthetic hormones," I told him. "I would actually like to replace the hormones that I have lost so far, and try to regulate my hormones to mimic the way they were when they were producing at optimum."

"That's impossible," he told me. "The drug companies know best, dear." I almost laughed in his face. "The drug companies know best?" I asked incredulously. That sounds ludicrous. The drug companies are a business—they don't have my best interests at heart. From my reading, I knew that the synthetic hormones recommended by these doctors are made from mares' urine and chemicals not found in the human body, and do nothing to replace the hormones we are no longer making naturally. I left his office vowing never to return, but where to go next? I had to start getting some sleep or I thought I would go crazy.

Then I heard about Dr. Schwarzbein, who, I found out, specialized in hormone replacement therapy. I thank the day I walked into her office. She understood what I was going through and reassured me that we were going to get my hormones in balance through replacement therapy and proper diet. Well, the diet was a snap for me, because it adhered to the principles of Somersizing. Her program, like mine, limits the intake of sugars to keep insulin levels balanced, while enjoying a delicious array of proteins, fats, and limited carbohydrates. Easy! I was already doing this.

"Now," she said, "the second part is a bit of a pain because we are going to track your hormonal levels, which requires you to have your blood levels checked regularly throughout the year." Also, because of the high-stress factor of my career, hormones tend to get out of balance more easily, because stress blocks estrogen receptors. When estrogen levels are lowered, you are more susceptible to weight gain and other symptoms of menopause. When I experienced a hot flash or any other symptom, it would be a sign that my hormonal balances were off, I was to call her and go over my stress levels, any change in my diet, or some significant life event that might be upsetting the delicate balance. If none of these factors was present, then a blood test would be required.

She started me on a regimen of *real* hormones that are plant based: estradiol, progesterone, and testosterone. These hormones are identical to the hormones found in the human body, as opposed to synthetic chemicals. The drug companies aren't interested in manufacturing natural hormones because you can't patent a natural substance, so they can't make a gazillion dollars off baby boomers going into menopause! Well, in a very short time, my husband, Alan, didn't know what had hit him. It was (and is) grand. I went from looking at him with irritation to looking at him and thinking, "Heeeey, big boy." I'm back with a vengeance sexually, but the real miracle is the sense of well-being and the good feelings I experience on a regular basis.

My sister has also suffered from hormone depletion. She couldn't sleep, was having hot flashes, and was experiencing short-term memory loss, loss of libido, and worst of all (for her) weight gain. Since Maureen is a breast cancer survivor, her doctors took her off all hormone replacement, because of the belief that estrogen supplements feed breast cancer. My sister is a beautiful woman. It just didn't seem fair that after having a mastectomy, surviving cancer, and being a faithful Somersizer, she could no longer take hormones and now had to endure these horrible side effects.

I recommended to my sister that she meet with Dr. Schwarzbein, because her thoughts about breast cancer and estrogen are contrary to common beliefs. Dr. Schwarzbein believes that it is an imbalance of hormones that creates an environment conducive to breast cancer, not just estrogen alone. Now Maureen is in the process of building up her natural hormones, though it has taken some time. According to Dr. Schwarzbein, you cannot give a woman who has zeroed out hormonally a full dose of hormones immediately. They must be replaced slowly, and monitored regularly. At first my sister reported she was gaining weight, but the

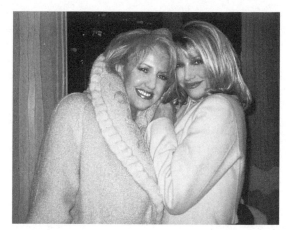

My sister Maureen and me.

weight was coming from increased bone mass. In other words, because her hormones had been completely depleted, her bones had become hollow, which is what happens in osteoporosis. Replacement therapy was balancing her hormones and building her bones. Getting in balance is a patience game. Now she is starting to lose the unwanted weight, realizing that it will take a little time to get her hormone levels back to normal. Even more important, she has a newfound sense of well-being and contentment, and the knowledge that she is creating a healthy environment of balanced hormones.

One thing I know for sure: when your hormones are not balanced, weight gain occurs. Whenever I see women of my age or older, I can tell which ones are on natural hormone replacement therapy and which are on synthetic hormones. I can tell by the areas of weight gain. Those taking no hormones or synthetic hormones struggle with big butt, bellies, thighs, neck, arms, and have a matronly look. Unfortunately, very few doctors have kept up with the latest findings and are uninformed of the benefits of actually *replacing* lost hormones. Most doctors try to impose synthetic hormones on their menopausal patients because they are easier. Most women are relieved to get this medication because the awful symptoms are alleviated. But *synthetic hormones do not replace lost hormones.* That is why most women on synthetic estrogen are gaining weight even though they might be eating perfectly. If you skipped over Dr. Schwarzbein's foreword and want further information on hormonal balance, I highly suggest you read it.

Without our hormones we die. That is what old age is about. When we are old, our bodies stop producing hormones that keep us alive. Even in our parents' and grandparents' time, the life span was shorter. As far as menopause, women were expected to simply endure and suffer through it. Those same women also did not have the stress associated with the lives we are living today. Women of previous generations were not in the workforce. Fatherless homes were a rarity. Pressures were less intense. Stress blocks estrogen receptors. Every time any of us goes through a stressful period of time, estrogen is blocked, which leaves us open to weight gain, and the accompanying factors associated with hormonal loss. Dr. Schwarzbein refers to this as "accelerated metabolic aging." In other words, the inner organs start to shut down from hormonal loss, which leaves us open to the diseases of the aged.

We trust that our doctors will keep up with the latest breakthroughs to handle this new phenomenon of living longer. It is said that we of this generation will live to be 100

years old on the average. I want those extra years to be glorious and healthy. Physicians who have not kept up with science and the latest breakthroughs are doing a disservice to their patients. Doctors need to stay informed of the latest studies, and give their patients the opportunity to choose what is best for them. Most doctors get all their "current information" only from drug companies who are trying to hawk their next multibillion-dollar drug. I can tell you from my own experience, I would never choose synthetic hormones. Real hormones keep us young on the outside as well as on the inside. Hormones protect us from the diseases of aging. Who wouldn't want that?

If you are struggling with symptoms of diminished hormones, you may be a candidate for hormone replacement therapy. If Somersizing is not working for you, and you can honestly say that you are following the program faithfully, then it is likely that you are in need of actual *natural* hormone replacement therapy. Check with your doctor. Now that I have my hormones balanced, I am enjoying this passage more than any other passage of my life so far, and my weight is under control and back to normal. I have wisdom, perspective, and contentment. My body is feeling young and supple. With hormones my thinking is sharp and sex is incredibly enjoyable because I am in the mood most of the time, without any worries about pregnancy.

This is a great time of life if you have the information to handle the changes inherent in your system. All I can tell you is that you don't have to suffer. I take my hormones gleefully every morning, calling them my "happy pills." This is what is working for me.

Because we are living longer than ever before, we need to approach the second half of our lives differently. Hormone replacement therapy is controversial. Some doctors feel adamant that estrogen is something to be taken in conservative doses. One doctor told me that she never recommends more than 2.00 milligrams of estrogen a day. In discussing this with Dr. Schwarzbein, she said that would be assuming that all women have the same chemical makeup. I am taking considerably more than that per day because that is what I require to keep my estrogen levels balanced. Everyone requires different amounts.

My body responds immediately to estrogen depletion. If I take my hormones two hours later than prescribed, I start to have symptoms. Usually it begins with an itch on my leg, or a small headache, or a heat comes over me. I am one of those women whose body requires a large and regular steady stream of estrogen divided into three supplements a day. I take my supplements every eight hours. Now, if Dr. Schwarzbein were to have a cap on estrogen dosage of 2 milligrams a day, regardless of my body's physiological requirements, I would not be enjoying the relief I get from my prescribed dosage. This is all new information and a new approach to replacement therapy. There are no conclusive studies to back up the effects. Yet I have chosen this approach because it is working for me. I feel great. I have energy and vigor, and seem to be aging more slowly than my peers. But if this were simply about looking good I would not take any substance that was potentially risky. I am enthused about hormone replacement therapy because I truly believe I will live longer and, most important, better, as a healthy person. I do not want to have to endure the diseases of old age if I can help it. If I am going to live longer, I want quality of life as well as quantity, and I hope you feel that way too.

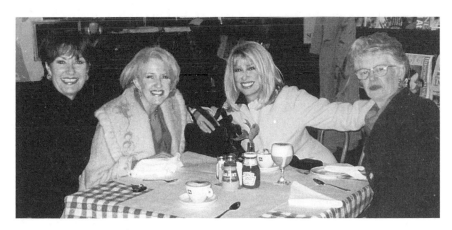

Our Birthday Club—my sister-in-law Mardi, my sister Maureen, and my Auntie Helen. We've been meeting for lunch for one another's birthdays for thirty-five years. Sadly, my mother is missing.

EIGHT

Somersizing for Children

My heart always goes out to overweight children, because other kids can be so mean. As if growing up isn't hard enough, I can only imagine how humiliating it is to bear the teasing and taunting from cruel youngsters. (Certainly many adults can be just as cruel!)

As always, check with your doctor before putting yourself or your children on any weight loss program. That being said, I have received many letters from parents thanking me for finally finding the solution to the problems of their overweight children. But Somersizing need not be reserved for overweight children. This is a smart and healthy way to eat for all children! Many people will say to me they couldn't possibly get their kids to eat this way. They only like white bread, American cheese, pizza, spaghetti, and McDonald's hamburgers and French fries. If this sounds like your child, these habits will be difficult to break. Your child has already developed an addiction to car-

bohydrates that will lead to an unhealthy pattern of eating and quite possibly a life-long struggle with weight.

We feed our children a diet of sugar. Cereal and milk for breakfast—sugar and sugar. Orange juice—sugar. A banana—sugar. For lunch we send them off with bologna sandwiches on white bread—sugar and sugar. A bag of chips—sugar. A box of juice—sugar. Snacks are cookies, candy, Popsicles, crackers, or chips—more sugar. For dinner we feed them macaroni and cheese—sugar. We pray they'll eat a single floret of broccoli, then we give them dessert—sugar.

Another problem for children these days is that they are leading sedentary lifestyles at an early age. Computer games, video games, and television have replaced physical activity for our youngsters. It is up to you! If you do not limit these activities, you are putting your child's health at risk. I know the TV and the computer can be great baby-sitters, but you must keep your children active. Get them involved in sports. Or get them to go out and "play." Remember when kids used to go out and "play"? Sadly, our streets and parks are not as safe as they once were, but you must find safe havens for your kids to get physical.

It's no wonder childhood obesity is on the rise! We no longer offer a piece of fruit for a snack—we give our children fruit roll-ups that are loaded with sugar and only remotely resemble fruit in its original form. Even healthy snacks, like yogurt, have been replaced with neon-colored and overly sugared substitutes that contain far more harm than good. Cookies and cakes used to be baked by Mom with fresh eggs, butter, sugar, and flour. Now our cookies and cakes aren't made with butter but with trans fats like partially hydrogenated oils plus a whole list of chemicals and preservatives! Our food supply is getting further and further away from real foods. If kids eat protein, it's often laden with sugar in the form of hot dogs, fast food burgers, and luncheon meats.

The sugar we feed our kids is poison. All this sugar causes an oversecretion of insulin. Our kids are filling up on sugar and their cells are becoming overloaded! As I've said, when the cells cannot handle any more sugar, the sugars and starches get converted to fat. This happens for kids as well as adults. I don't mean to place blame, because most people don't know how bad sugar and starch can be, but if you are feeding your child a diet of sugar you must begin now to reverse the process.

Children learn to eat the foods we expose them to. They learn to want "kiddie foods" because that's what we give them when they are very young, thinking they need plain, bland foods at a young age. You do not need to make separate meals for your kids, if you train them at an early age to like the taste of real food. My grandchildren are a fascinating example. (I know what you're thinking . . . another overzealous grandmother who's going to bore me with a "listen how wonderful my grandchildren are" story. Sorry, you're right!) Alan and I now have five grandchildren and all of them are terrific eaters. Daisy comes to my house and begs for my delicious fennel soup. One of Ziane's favorite lunches is a plate of fresh tomatoes, stinky French cheese, and sardines. Camelia loves green beans, sautéed wild mushrooms, and Parmesan cheese. Baby Violet, not yet two, asks to nibble on blue cheese while sitting in the grocery cart. She was at our house the other day and I offered her some cheddar cheese. She said, "No Zannie, I want Brie." She even likes celery with vinaigrette!

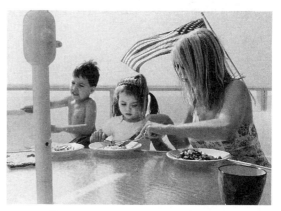

Somersizers in training . . . my grandchildren.

Children eat the foods you start them on. I never made my son, Bruce, eat "kid food." He always loved my cooking and ate whatever I made him. At five his favorite meal was steamed clams. I remember on his birthday I took him to Scoma's in Sausalito for his favorite dinner—steamed clams. I had so little money at the time. I was a single mother struggling to get by. Fortunately, I'd just gotten a modeling job, so I had a few dollars to treat him to this special birthday meal. We ordered one bowl of steamed clams after another, dipping them into garlic and butter. Our faces were covered with butter and smiles. I looked down in my wallet to make sure I had enough money for a slice of cheesecake for dessert and a tip for the wait-

ress. Bruce was beaming with happiness. He has always been the greatest joy of my life.

When our wonderful evening came to a close I asked the waitress for the bill. She told me that a gentleman across the room watched us eat our dinner and said he had never seen two people enjoy their dinner more. He paid the tab and left anonymously. To this day I still do not know the identity of this kind stranger, but I'll never forget that magical night with Bruce.

Back to my point, if you start them on steamed clams, they might just love them! If they don't like it the first time, don't assume they never will. Keep letting them taste things. Often they will acquire a taste as time goes by. Why do you think Dr. Seuss

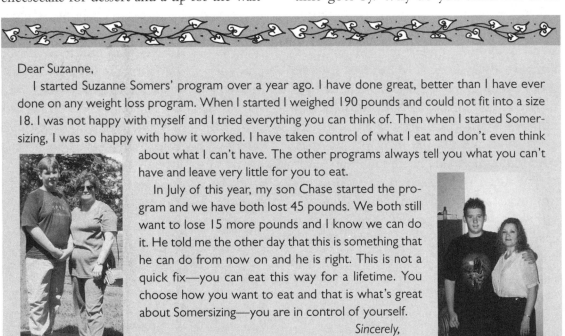

Dear Suzanne,

I started Suzanne Somers' program over a year ago. I have done great, better than I have ever done on any weight loss program. When I started I weighed 190 pounds and could not fit into a size 18. I was not happy with myself and I tried everything you can think of. Then when I started Somersizing, I was so happy with how it worked. I have taken control of what I eat and don't even think about what I can't have. The other programs always tell you what you can't have and leave very little for you to eat.

In July of this year, my son Chase started the program and we have both lost 45 pounds. We both still want to lose 15 more pounds and I know we can do it. He told me the other day that this is something that he can do from now on and he is right. This is not a quick fix—you can eat this way for a lifetime. You choose how you want to eat and that is what's great about Somersizing—you are in control of yourself.

Sincerely,
Lois S. Fossitt

before

after

wrote *Green Eggs and Ham?* How many children will say, "No, no, no, I don't like that," when they have never even tried it! You must be "Sam I Am" and *insist* until they do. Who knows . . . they may like it on a box and with a fox, they may like it here or there. They may like it everywhere! Bruce and his wife, Caroline, started a family rule that the kids have to taste one bite of new foods. More than half the time, Camelia will go from saying, "I don't like that," to "Mommy, I *do* like it!"

If you start them early on McDonald's, that's what they'll ask for. How many times have I heard people say, "He just won't eat anything else! I've tried and tried." Believe me, your children will not starve if you don't give in to their junk food cravings. Again, it starts young. Violet loves her bites of chicken, broccoli, and brown rice, but the first time she tasted a peanut butter and jelly sandwich she flipped! Let's face it, sugar tastes good! Even a baby can recognize that. After Violet had her first taste of PB & J she started asking for it frequently. We love our kids and of course we want to give them whatever they ask for. My daughter-in-law, Caroline, knows the dangers of too much sugar so she stopped feeding Violet peanut butter and jelly (except on rare occasions). You see how the patterns begin. The baby tastes something sweet and wonderful. Then she continues asking for it around every turn. At first Caroline gave it to her, but then it became a habit. Violet was pushing away her dinner of meat, vegetables, and whole grains and asking for peanut butter and jelly. Caroline felt she had to break the habit before Violet turned off healthier options.

Caroline's solution was . . . let her cry! Let her have a big ol' tantrum and throw her body down on the ground, chanting over and over, "I wan a peanut budder and sangwich!" Caroline would look at her very calmly and say, "Violet, I know you want peanut butter and jelly, but we're not going to have that for dinner tonight." And she'd present her with a lovely meal made up of *real* foods, like bites of steak, steamed green beans, and whole wheat pasta tossed in butter and Parmesan cheese. Now Violet eats peanut butter and jelly occasionally and is back to loving her meats, exotic cheeses, whole-grain carbohydrates, fresh fruit, and vegetables. By the way, if you *are* going to give kids peanut butter and jelly, make the sandwich on whole-grain bread and use sugarless peanut butter (like Laura Scudder's) and all-fruit jam. At least the effects of insulin will be lessened.

The solution is to keep your children's exposure to sugar and highly starchy foods to a minimum. Most kids will greatly benefit from Somersizing on Level Two, where they will enjoy a combination of proteins, fats,

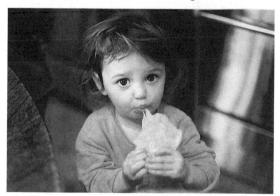

Yum! A mango pit! My granddaughter hasn't discovered white sugar yet.

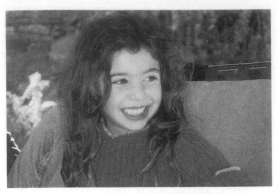

My darling granddaughter.

vegetables low in starch, whole-grain carbohydrates, and fresh fruit. In addition, I think a good general rule is to try to limit them to one sugary treat a day (one piece of candy, a bowl of ice cream, a piece of birthday cake, a Popsicle, a fruit roll-up, etc.). It's unrealistic to completely eliminate sugar from your child's diet. (Although many people do this with success.) When you start them young, they learn to monitor themselves. This is exactly what has happened with Camelia. She's only four and already she has good eating habits. She spent the night last week and I offered her a bowl of ice cream after dinner. She said, "But I already had a cupcake at school today because it was Juliette's birthday." Truth be told, I gave her a small bowl anyway, because it was a special night with Zannie, but I loved the fact that she has her sugar intake in check.

Don't misunderstand my advice. I don't want you to become militant with your kids. And I especially don't believe in withholding desserts as a punishment, because I worry it can lead to an obsession with food, which could later result in eating disorders. I remember a very prissy girl from grade school whom I'll call Merry Beth. I went to her house to play, and her kitchen cabinets were locked so that she couldn't sneak any food! We were only in fourth grade and I couldn't believe she was not allowed to eat unless her mother approved it. Many years later, prissy little Merry Beth had become an overweight promiscuous teen. She bleached her hair blond and wore the shortest skirts in town. It seems possible that her acting out was a result of a controlling mother who probably thought she was helping her child by locking the food away. This is how we become obsessed with the forbidden fruit! Please, expose your child to healthy food to avoid these problems, but let them have a little fun too.

Many people *think* they are feeding their children a healthy diet, when this couldn't be further from the truth. I was at the house of a friend who has struggled with her weight for years. We were talking about the importance of good eating habits for health reasons, not for vanity reasons. We were talking about the importance of real foods, like meat, fish, and fresh vegetables. She looked me straight in the face and told me she eats plenty of vegetables and salads. I have never seen any vegetables other than iceberg lettuce in her refrigerator! And she covers it in fat-free bottled dressing filled with chemicals, sugar, and starchy fillers! If you eat out of bottles, cans, jars, and boxes, you are not a healthy eater! If you eat a lot of sandwiches and pasta you are not a healthy eater! If your idea of vegetables is iceberg lettuce, you are not a healthy eater! If you feed your family a meal made up mostly of starch, you are not a healthy eater!

It starts with you . . . the parents. If your child already has bad eating habits, if your entire family already has bad eating habits, then you will have to retrain everyone to eat properly. It may not be as hard as you think. Children love great-tasting food. If they reject it at first, don't give up. They are detoxing from sugar! They will lose the cravings for sugar once it is greatly reduced in their diets. I read from a child development expert that you must attempt a new food with a child 200 times before they might accept it! The key is not to give them a lot. Just one little piece of broccoli to start. This turnaround is possible and it may be the greatest gift you ever give to your children. Help them develop healthy habits that will keep them trim and vital, especially if obesity runs in the family. Be a role model. I know you do not want your children to suffer the painful realities of being overweight. Get the whole family on the path to healthy eating.

It's easier to accomplish this if you can make dinner a time to gather as a family, a time where you can be thankful for the good food you are eating and a time to share your day with each other. One of the many things I admire about Alan's son, Stephen, is how he and his wife, Olivia, make mealtime a family ritual. Every night, they gather around the table with their two beautiful boys and enjoy a delicious meal. Ziane is now five and he loves his new baby brother, Becket. Becket is our fifth grandchild. What a darling baby! He's so calm and happy. Stephen and Olivia are exceptional parents and wonderful cooks. Stephen's coq au vin is one of the best I've ever tasted. Olivia is a whiz when it comes to desserts. They derive great joy out of creating delicious food. Ziane has more energy than any child I know! Still, they make sure that he sits down for dinner without the distractions of the television or other toys. They truly cherish this sacred family time around the table. Don't tell me your child has a hard time sitting still and must eat dinner on the run, or in his room in front of the TV. You, the parents, make the rules of the house and if you enforce them, they become family *traditions,* rather than family rules.

I hope you'll make Somersizing a family event. You and your children will greatly benefit from eating real, healthy, delicious foods while gathered together around a family table.

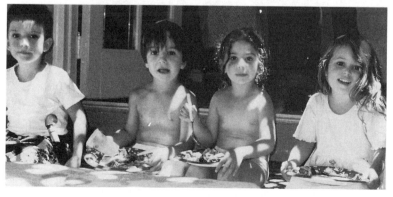

We connect through meals, even the grandchildren.

A NEW YEAR, A FRESH START

New Year's is an obvious time to make some changes regarding your lifestyle. We all want to start the year fresh and make our minds and our bodies the best they can be. Last year, when we celebrated not only a new year but a new century and a new millennium, Alan and I talked at great length about how we would celebrate. We had an offer to fly around the world to celebrate the millennium in every time zone. We were invited to Israel to party in a bedouin tent placed in the middle of the desert and surrounded by camels. We had friends who wanted us to join them in South Africa. I had opportunities to perform at numerous casinos and parties.

When it came right down to it, we decided to celebrate this important evening with our children. Leslie, Frank, Stephen, Olivia, Bruce, and Caroline all came to Palm Springs for a New Year's feast. We spent the day swimming and playing with the five grandchildren. I fed the kids their dinner early and they went to bed at a reasonable hour (except Camelia, who was determined to stay up until midnight! She fell asleep on the couch during the salad course). We all dressed up in our fancy clothes and I prepared a rather outstanding meal. We began with the

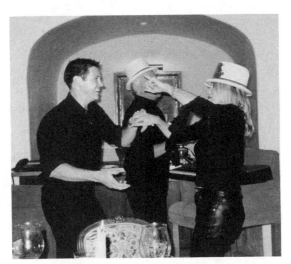

New Year's Eve 2000—dancing with my son, Bruce.

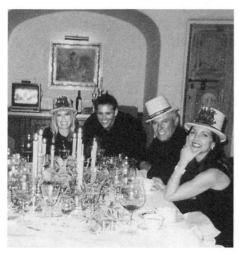

New Year's Eve 2000—
after the party.

finest caviar and French champagne. Decadence was definitely in order to ring in the year 2000! Our salad was a butter lettuce salad with sliced fennel, shaved truffles, and toasted pine nuts. It was then dressed with olive oil, truffle oil, and lemon juice. For our entrée, I prepared tenderloin of beef with rich brown sauce, accompanied by puréed celery root and fresh asparagus. On a night like that, you save room for dessert because it was worth it. I made awesome chocolate soufflés with chocolate sauce and freshly whipped cream.

Even more spectacular than the food was the connection we had as a family. The intimacy we shared that night is a treasure none of us will ever forget. There were no sloppy drunks standing too close and yelling in our ears. There were no unwanted kisses shared at the stroke of midnight. There was no worrying about driving on the most dangerous night of the year. We danced and laughed and sang in the year 2000. We watched the telecast from around the world—awed by the spectacular Eiffel Tower fireworks display, and even our own little show in Palm Springs.

Little Camelia woke up just after midnight. I held her tightly as we watched the fireworks light up the night sky. I told her that all her life people will ask where she was on New Year's 2000, and just as I will remember, she will say she was at the most special place in the world . . . at home with her family.

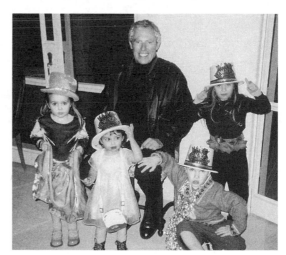

Alan and the grandchildren.

Taking Control of Your Life

Our job as adults is complicated. It is up to us individually to become thoroughly familiarized with those idiosyncrasies particular to our own bodies. If caffeine wreaks havoc with you chemically, stop drinking caffeine. If sugar gives you horrible mood swings and PMS, stop eating sugar. If body image is important to you and you have a weight problem, get help to understand what foods your body can handle. In other words, our chemicals should not be controlling us, we should control our chemicals. Don't let yourself be put in a position of powerlessness because you were too lazy to handle your body's needs. If it is as simple as finding what works for your body, why not do it?

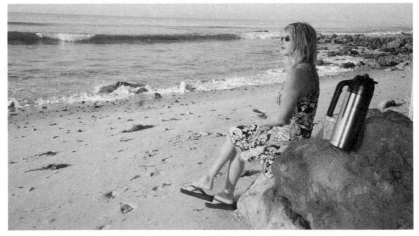

Morning light: first cup of decaf.

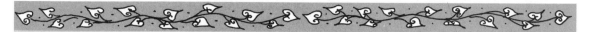

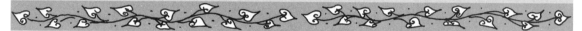

If you are addicted to food, it is important to know that at the heart of every addiction lies an anesthetized old hurt looking for a way to be released. Addictions are never about being hungry, or thirsty, or needing to have more "things." Addictions are distractions from pain. Pain comes from an inability to tell the truth to yourself about what has happened to you, in your past or present. We become addicted because we do not want to face the truth about our life or its effects upon us. Accepting the painful truth, rather than running from it, is the beginning of healing. Nothing less succeeds. Healing yourself requires admitting some old hurt. The anger you have spent your life trying to conceal comes not because you have done something bad, but because you have been emotionally injured.

Once you can accept that truth, it will become easier for you to continue facing other truths about yourself. I have spent most of my adult life working at facing those issues I have used as excuses for not trying. Facing the truth about myself has been the single most valuable thing I have ever done for my self-esteem. I believe doing this "work," and experiencing the peace that has accompanied it, is the basis for my happiness. Do your best to understand the effects of the pain in your life. When you can tell yourself the truth at every opportunity, you will be on the path to healing those things you've been carrying around for so long. In time you will find that relief does not come from what is inside your refrigerator, but from being totally honest with yourself.

It is in your own best interests to heal yourself by being honest about what has hurt you in your life. When you can find that answer, healing will begin, and you will no longer need to look at a cookie as a substitute. You are in control of changing your thinking, your attitude, and your body shape. People are always telling me they want to lose weight and change their life. Unfortunately, wanting to change the course of your life, or lose that extra weight you've been carrying around for the past while, is not enough. "Wanting" is not an active state of being. It involves living in the future, not in the present where you can actually do the work to make what you "want" a reality. Losing weight and creating a happier life requires commitment.

You must *commit* to starting the program right now, this minute, or else you will always find a reason for postponing. It's hard to find the appropriate words that will explain how freeing this eating experience is going to be for you. The food is truly delicious, and once you start losing weight you will forget that this loss came as a result of changing the way you now approach food. Once you understand the effects of sugar and the havoc it creates on your hormonal system, you really start to think about it every time you ingest sugar. After a while, sugary foods fall into a category of "is it really worth it?" And, I might add, some-

times these foods are worth it—sometimes I really want that plate of fresh, hot, crisp French fries. But there's a difference now. In the past, I used to gobble up platefuls of fries and chips without thinking about the effects of excess carbohydrates on my physiology; now, I do think about it. And the question always comes up—is it worth it? Is it worth messing with my newly reprogrammed metabolism by raising my insulin levels, which will lead to weight gain? More often than not, when I think it through, I end up pushing the cake, or pie, or fries away.

It's your life. This program has helped me to look at food once again as my friend. I look forward to mealtimes. I am never hungry, and I am in control of my weight. I *committed* to this program and the weight went away. As long as I continue to eat the Somersize way, I know I can happily maintain my ideal body composition.

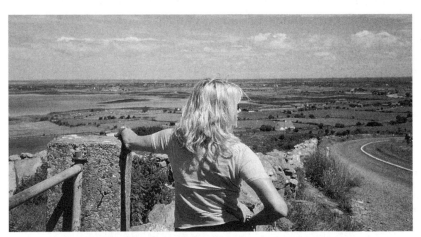

Discovering my Irish roots, overlooking Galway Bay.

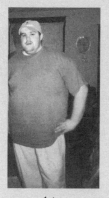

before

Dear Suzanne,

I would like to take this opportunity to say thank you, your program has helped me so much. I have tried many diets before, with little or no success. Then last October, a friend of mine was reading your book, *Get Skinny on Fabulous Food*. She was telling me about it, but I was very skeptical, since most of the programs that I had tried before revolved around eliminating the fats from your diet in order to lose weight. No offense, but after reviewing your diet plan, I thought you were "nuts!" My friend, Courtney, explained what your book says about the way that we digest fats and proteins, so I thought that I would give the diet a try. So I started on a Monday morning, which gave me the weekend to buy the proper foods and get my mind set. I found it kind of hard at first, since my body was so used to the snacks and junk food that I had been giving it. But, I must say that it wasn't as hard as I expected, and after a few days, the cravings were less and less. I lost 8 pounds the first week, which motivated me to keep going.

The more weight that has come off, the more my self-esteem has gone up. The only exercise that I have been doing on a regular basis is walking. I was very impressed with my willpower when I was able to get through Thanksgiving and Christmas without giving in to temptation even once! I will admit that I do have "Funky Foods," but I always keep them in moderation. My friends say that I am an inspiration to them, and my family has told me how proud they are of me—that kind of praise makes me feel really good about myself. The thing that makes me feel the best though, is that I have been able to buy clothes in much smaller sizes. Sometimes I have trouble believing that it's all true, that in less than one year I have lost 124 pounds!

I have always hated physical exercise, but since I have lost the weight, I have a lot more energy, and after doing my walking or whatever, I feel really good. I would like to lose another 50 pounds, although my mom thinks I look really good right now (she doesn't want me to get too skinny). Now that I have lost enough to be able to work out, I am hinting for a gym membership for my Christmas present.

I just want to thank you again for your time and your help. I have told those around me that you are a Godsend, and I truly believe that. You have helped me so much and I thank you from the bottom of my heart. I hope that you will continue to help the overweight people out there who have given up hope of finding something that will work for them. You are my angel—that is the only way that I can describe what you mean to me!

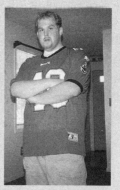

after

Yours respectfully,
Jody Love

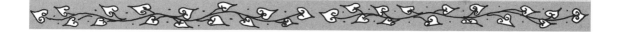

Taking Control of Your Life

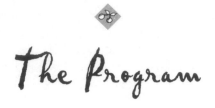

TEN

The Program

Now that we've covered why Somersizing works and you understand how crucial it is to balance our hormones, let's get down to the nuts and bolts of what you eat on a day-to-day basis.

ELIMINATE

As we've discussed, the most important foods to eliminate are the ones that cause our blood sugar to fluctuate too much. In addition to sugar and white flour, I have made a list of Funky Foods that cause similar problems.

The first group of Funky Foods is made up of sugar sources. Some are natural and some are refined, but natural or not, they're still sugar and I avoid them completely when I'm trying to lose weight.

SUGARS

White sugar	Molasses
Brown sugar	Honey
Raw sugar	Maple syrup
Corn syrup	Beets
Sucrose	Carrots

I know it seems weird to eliminate carrots, which have many nutritional qualities, including essential beta carotene and Vitamin A, but carrots are very high in sugar and we get plenty of beta carotene from broccoli and kale, and Vitamin A is found in cantaloupe, peaches, and apricots.

The next group of Funky Foods is made up of foods high in starch. These turn directly to sugar (glucose) upon digestion. And remember, we don't need to give our bodies extra sugar, because we can burn our fat reserves for energy instead.

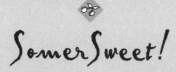

SomerSweet!

For ten years I've been looking for the miracle sweetener that would allow me to enjoy the taste of sugar without the harmful effects of insulin or the chemical effects of artificial sweeteners. Millions of people consume aspartame (NutraSweet, Equal) in large amounts without realizing its dangerous effects. I have read far too many controversial reports on the dangers of this chemical sweetener. It has been reported that more than 80% of all food additive complaints to the FDA are related to aspartame. Additionally, I have read frightening studies reporting that aspartame has been known to cause irreversible brain damage in laboratory animals. One can of diet soda may be enough to raise the toxins in an infant's brain higher than levels that damaged brains of immature lab animals. We must eliminate this chemical from our lives!

In my last book, I told you about an all-natural sweetener called stevia, which was better than sugar or chemicals, but had a bitter aftertaste and was difficult to incorporate into recipes. I even included a few recipes with saccharin, so that you could enjoy the taste of something sweet, but I warned you about overeating this chemical sweetener. Even new Spenda is chemically based. There must be a better alternative!

Now all my prayers have been answered with SomerSweet. SomerSweet is a natural, sweet fiber that is 99.9% chemical free! It's sugar-free, so it won't spike insulin, and each serving has less than 1 gram of carbohydrate! This is the most exciting breakthrough in all my years of Somersizing. Now I can offer you something to stir in your coffee or tea, sprinkle on your cereal, and to make fabulous Level One desserts! It's truly a miracle.

SomerSweet is a blend of fiber, fructose and soy extract to create a low glycemic, delicious product. Fiber—you know, it's the stuff your body needs anyway! In fact, the proprietary fiber in SomerSweet helps feed the good bacteria in your intestine, which keeps you healthy and also keeps you regular! It's the fiber your body needs with the flavor your taste buds crave. This fiber is then blended with a special type of fructose—a natural sweetener which has a minimal effect on blood sugar. In fact, SomerSweet causes such a modest insulin response, it's even safe for diabetics and approved by the French Diabetics Associ-

(continued on next page)

ation! On the glycemic index, fructose is about 20. To give you a comparison, that's about the same as snow peas.

Since SomerSweet does not create a significant insulin response, you can use this wonderful, sweet, natural fiber instead of sugar or chemical sweeteners and still lose weight! Plus, unlike sugar, SomerSweet will not get you started on sugar binges that keep you craving sweets all day long. You'll enjoy an incredible serving of one of my rich and delicious desserts and feel satisfied. You won't be headed back to the kitchen an hour later during your sugar crash looking for more sweets!

Perhaps the most exciting news about SomerSweet is that it's great for baking! You can bake it, broil it, fry it, freeze it, and re-heat it and it still remains stable! I have never found a substitute for sugar that works so well in baking. Now you really can have your cake and eat it, too! It even caramelizes to make toppings for crème brûlée!

You'll find several recipes that include SomerSweet in this book, like Vanilla Bean and Chocolate Ice Cream, Raspberry Soufflé, Light Chocolate Mousse, and Molten Chocolate Cakes. Plus, look for my Somersize Dessert book, in November 2001 for thirty new, sinful recipes made exclusively with SomerSweet!

It's SomerSweet—a natural fiber with a miraculous, sweet taste. Sugar free! 99.9% chemical free! No aftertaste! Great for baking! Low calorie! Low carbohydrate! Low glycemic index! Safe for diabetics! It's a miracle.

SomerSweet is coming soon to stores and is now available at SuzanneSomers.com.

STARCHES

White flour	Yams
White rice	Pumpkin
Corn	Butternut squash
Potatoes	Acorn squash
Sweet potatoes	Hubbard squash
Parsnips	Bananas

There are so many wonderful alternatives to white flour: whole wheat, pumpernickel, rye, amaranth, spelt, and kamut to name a few. White rice can be replaced with brown rice, which has a wonderful earthy flavor, or, better yet, wild rice, which has even less starch. As for corn and potatoes, you will be eating greater amounts of green vegetables rather than filling up on starchy vegetables, which cause a sugar surge and extra pounds. Think about the fact that corn and potatoes are most often used to fatten up our livestock and then maybe it won't be so hard to resist that plate of fries! And I know you will be shocked when I tell you to eliminate bananas—how about all that potassium? Sorry, but bananas are very high in sugar and with all the other fruits you can eat, you won't miss them.

The third group of Funky Foods doesn't

seem to fit into any of our four Somersize Food Groups because these foods contain protein or fat *and* carbohydrates. Take nuts: they are a protein, they do have fat, *and* they are rich in carbohydrates. That makes them a no-no for Somersizing purposes. Of all the Funky Foods, the foods on this list are the least of your problems. When you graduate to Level Two, these are the first foods you may incorporate back into your meals. In fact, many eat olives, avocado, and soy products on Level One and still enjoy all the effects of losing weight and feeling great. I regularly eat edamame (the green vegetable form of soybeans) without any problems. They are a great source of protein and fat, and even though they have a little carbohydrate, I find that eating them does not disrupt my weight loss. Plus, they are so good for you!

BAD COMBO FOODS

Nuts	Soy
Olives	Low-fat or whole milk
Liver	Low-fat or full fat soy milk
Avocados	Low-fat or full fat rice milk
Coconuts	Buttermilk

The last group of Funky Foods is made up of caffeine and alcohol. Just like other Funky Foods, caffeine can cause highs and lows in your blood sugar, which leads to insulin resistance. I'd hate to see you eat a perfectly combined meal and then blow it with one cup of coffee. Feel free to drink decaffeinated coffee (try Starbucks' delicious Guatemalan decaf) and herbal teas. And don't worry, when you combine correctly you'll have a steady source of energy to get you through the day, rather than experiencing the highs and lows that keep us reaching

for caffeine or sweets. As for alcohol, everyone knows it makes you fat, especially beer and hard liquor. Now that you understand the connection between insulin and weight gain around the midsection, a "beer belly" makes perfect sense. Red wine has recently been found to have beneficial effects and we will incorporate it later on when we are maintaining our weight, but during Level One we will steer clear of all alcohol. I do, however, make an exception with regard to cooking. If you are doing well on Level One you may use wine in some of my recipes because the alcohol burns off and it leaves a delicious flavor in your cooking.

CAFFEINE & ALCOHOL

Coffee	Beer
Caffeinated teas	Hard alcohol
Caffeinated sodas	
Cocoa (including unsweetened cocoa)	

I know it seems like a strange list of foods to eliminate, but soon it will become second nature. Sugar, starches, bad combo foods, caffeine, and alcohol are all avoided *completely* on Level One. But don't worry, you don't have to say good-bye to these foods forever. They'll be back, in moderation, when we reach our goal weight and advance to Level Two, the maintenance portion of Somersizing.

SEPARATE

In order to learn how to combine our foods in a way that maximizes our digestion, we must first separate foods into our four Somersize categories: Proteins/Fats, Carbos,

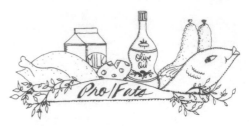

Veggies, and Fruits. Although many foods are made up of a combination of protein, fat, and carbohydrate, we have grouped them by their predominant feature to help simplify the program. For instance, *all* the foods found in the Carbos, Veggies, and Fruits groups contain carbohydrates, but the carbohydrate levels vary greatly, which is why I have broken them down into different groups. I have briefly described each group here, and have included complete lists of these foods in the Appendix, which you'll find at the back of the book.

Pro/Fats

The first Somersize group is made up of foods high in protein and/or fat. I put these two food groups together because many of the foods that contain protein also contain fat. Meat, poultry, fish, eggs, cheese, butter, and cream are just a few of the Pro/Fats you'll enjoy.

Proteins are made up of organic compounds called amino acids. These amino acids are the building blocks for the human body. Proteins play a role in virtually every cellular function: they regulate muscle contraction, antibody production, and blood vessel expansion and contraction to main-

THE CONNECTION BETWEEN CAFFEINE AND COMFORT FOODS

When you drink caffeine, you increase your adrenaline. Oh, how we love that caffeine rush in the morning, at lunchtime, or during that afternoon dip. But increased adrenaline blocks estrogen receptors and increases insulin levels. Since insulin is the fat-storing hormone, we don't want to drink caffeine with a meal because the insulin released could send the whole meal to the fat reserves. Also, caffeine initially increases serotonin, which is called the "feel-good hormone," but then makes it lower over time. Low serotonin levels can trigger us to crave "comfort foods." Comfort foods vary from person to person, but usually they are high in carbohydrates (mashed potatoes, macaroni and cheese, cookies, cake, etc.). These comfort foods cause spikes in your insulin, and by now we all know the ill effects of raised insulin levels. Plus, caffeine raises adrenaline, and adrenaline breaks down lean body tissue. Lean body tissue is proportional to your metabolism. The less lean body mass, the lower your metabolism, which leaves you open to weight gain. It's hard to kick the habit at first, but I tell you, decaffeinated coffee is the way to go.

tain normal blood pressure. Protein is a critically important part of the diet because it supplies us with new amino acids that are needed to make these different proteins.

By now you understand the virtues of fat and know that completely eliminating fat from your diet is unhealthy. Fats provide a major storage form of metabolic fuel. When they break down they provide us energy. Fats also help to facilitate the use of essential fat-soluble vitamins like A, D, E, and K. Vitamin A is necessary for healthy eyes and skin; Vitamin D helps to absorb calcium; Vitamin E prevents cholesterol deposits; and Vitamin K contributes to healthy blood clotting. Fat also helps to stabilize blood sugar. And fat is the body's fuel source that causes the least amount of insulin response. Essential fatty acids cannot be manufactured by our bodies on their own; they, too, must be included in our daily meals. Unsaturated fats, like olive oil, canola oil, and fish oils, help to lower cholesterol levels and should be included in our meals.

Any of the foods in the Pro/Fats group can be eaten together, or in combination with Veggies. (See the complete list of Pro/Fats on pp. 267–268.)

Carbos

Carbohydrates are mostly derived from plant sources, rather than from animal sources. Carbos are the primary metabolic fuel in our westernized diets. As I explained earlier, carbos break down into glucose, which is one of the body's main sources of energy. (The other is fat.) Since we have other mechanisms in our bodies to produce

glucose, carbos are the one nutrient that is not absolutely essential in our diet.

Completely eliminating carbohydrates from our diet is dangerous. On the Somersize system we eliminate *refined* carbohydrates like sugar, white flour, and white rice, but we do enjoy complex carbohydrates, like whole-grain pastas and cereals, which still have many essential vitamins and nutrients intact. In addition, complex carbohydrates provide fiber and roughage necessary for the digestive process.

On an emotional level, carbohydrates cause a release of serotonin—the feel-good hormone. If you are prone to depression, completely eliminating carbohydrates causes a halt in serotonin levels, which can lead to depression. Be careful, however, of loading up on the wrong kinds of carbohydrates if you are depressed and looking for a serotonin fix. "Comfort foods," like macaroni and cheese or a turkey pot pie, may give you the serotonin release, but they also bring the ill effects of poorly combined, high-starch meals. Stick to reasonable amounts of the foods listed in Carbos group and you shouldn't have a problem.

Any of the foods in the Carbos group can be eaten together, or in combination with Veggies. (See the complete list of Carbos on p. 268.)

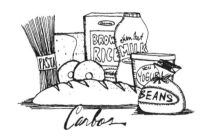

Many people ask me if you can Somersize if you are a vegetarian. The answer really depends on how strict you are. If you are the type of person who simply does not eat red meat, you will have no problem following the Level One guidelines. You can get plenty of protein and fat sources from poultry, fish, eggs, and dairy products.

If you do not eat any animal products, you will have a difficult time on Level One, because the only foods left in the Pro/Fats group are vegetable-based oils. This means you will be eating predominantly Carbos meals. Since carbos are not eaten with fats on Level One, I worry you will not get the essential fatty acids you need. Therefore, if you do not eat animal products, you should Somersize on Level Two. This way you can enjoy fats with your Carbos and Veggies meals. This is probably how you eat anyway, but you will eliminate the sugar and high-starch vegetables, and you will replace white flour, rice, bread, and pasta with their whole-grain counterparts. Anyone will benefit from making that simple change.

In addition, if you are a strict vegetarian and you need additional protein sources, I do make an exception regarding soy. Although tofu has protein, fat, and carbohydrates, I recommend you include it in your meals, either as a Pro/Fat or a Carbo (since it has protein, fat, and carbohydrate). As for soy milk, buy fat-free soy milk and treat it as a Carbo with the other nonfat dairy products.

Veggies

All vegetables are technically carbohydrates, but those found in this Somersize category have been chosen because they are low in starch and cause only a minute rise in the blood sugar. These include green beans, broccoli, cauliflower, artichokes, tomatoes, peppers, onions, and more. Vegetables are packed with vitamins and minerals and provide essential roughage for proper elimination. I implore you, fill up on vegetables! They are an essential part of your daily diet.

Any of the foods in the Veggies group can be eaten together. And since Veggies can easily be digested with either Pro/Fats *or* Carbos, you may eat them with either group. (See the complete list of Veggies on p. 269.)

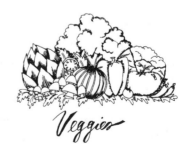

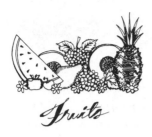

Fruits

Fruits

Fruits are also technically carbohydrates, but because of their unique sugar content, fruit must always be eaten alone. Fruits are a great source of fiber and help to keep the digestive tract moving. They are loaded with nutrients and vitamins, but if you mix fruit with other foods, it can lose its nutritional benefits and upset the digestive process. Fruit turns to acid when combined with other food groups and spoils in the stomach, causing gas and that horrible bloated feeling. Fruit as a supposedly "healthy" option for dessert can ruin a perfectly combined meal. Not only will it make you feel uncomfortable, but it can trap the energy of other foods and cause unnecessary storage of fat. So eat fruit . . . please eat fruit. But eat it alone to get the maximum benefits.

As far as fruit juice is concerned, most of the vital nutrients have been pressed out of the fruit by the time it is turned into juice. The remaining juice is mostly fruit sugar. Therefore, I recommend you eat the whole fruit to receive the fiber and drink fruit juice sparingly. Concentrated fruit juice is often used as a sugar substitute. Unfortunately, your body reacts exactly the same to fruit sugar as it does to regular sugar, because it makes your insulin spike. Every

ASPARAGUS—THE ALKALINE VEGETABLE

Many health care professionals feel that we are facing the most dangerous crisis in history. There have been numerous studies linking illness and disease to overacidity in our bodies. We want our bodies to be alkaline, not acidic. Unfortunately, we breathe polluted air, our food and water supply is filled with chemicals, and our stress levels are through the roof. All of these factors cause our bodies to overproduce acid wastes, which can upset the delicate alkaline-acid balance.

For more information on this serious health issue, I highly recommend you read Dr. Theodore A. Baroody's book, Alkalize or Die. *It gives important guidelines for evaluating your alkaline-acid situation, and how to fix it. One great way to reduce the acid in your body is to eat asparagus! Baroody cites asparagus as a powerful acid reducer and a known therapy for cancer. Its high ammonia content literally plummets your body into alkalinity in a short period of time. And it tastes great, too!*

Now when I go to pick my vegetable for my meals, I choose asparagus several times a week. I especially like it steamed and dipped in lemon dill mayonnaise.

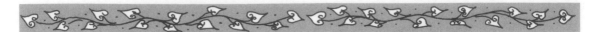

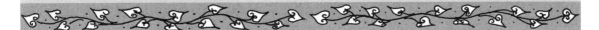

now and then I may have an all-fruit-juice-sweetened sorbet or Popsicle (on Level One), but not with great frequency, because in Level One we are trying to heal our insulin resistance. The same goes for dried fruit; the sugar concentration becomes far more intense with dried fruits. I eat them rarely, if at all, on Level One.

Here are some guidelines on how you can eat delicious and nutritious fresh fruit and gain all the benefits without creating digestion problems.

Eat Fruit on an empty stomach.

Eat Fruit alone, then wait twenty minutes, and you may follow up with a Carbos meal. (The twenty-minute lead time gets the digestion of the fruit going and eliminates problem combinations.)

Eat fruit alone, then wait one hour, and you may follow up with a Pro/Fats meal.

If you want Fruit for a snack or for dessert, you must wait two hours after your last meal to avoid any problems.

Any of the foods in the Fruit group can be eaten together. (See the complete list of Fruits on p. 269.)

Free Foods

There are a few items that may be combined with Pro/Fats, Veggies, or Carbos because they do not conflict with any of the food groups. These include soy sauce, vinegar, mustard, gelatin, herbs and spices. In addition, lemons and limes, though technically fruits, are very low in sugar and therefore may be used to flavor any of the four food groups.

The Glycemic Index

All carbohydrates will break down into sugar upon digestion. But, as we've discussed, some carbohydrates create a much larger insulin response than others. Although I do not ask you to calculate calories, fat grams, sugars, or even carbohydrates as part of the Somersize program, I am including this chart, called the Glycemic Index, to assist you in seeing the effects of various kinds of carbohydrates. The glycemic index rises corresponding to the level of hyperglycemia caused by eating carbohydrates. The higher the glycemic index, the higher the level of hyperglycemia.

You will notice that foods in their natural state have a lower glycemic index than foods that have been processed. Whole wheat bread breaks down into less glucose than its processed counterpart, white bread. Brown rice has a lower glycemic index than its refined counterpart, white rice. This is largely due to the fiber content of foods. The greater the fiber, the lower the glycemic index.

Fruits and vegetables are also carbohydrates, with varying degrees of glucose potential. Seeing how they rate on the glycemic index will help to explain how I divided all food into my four Somersize Food Groups. Those vegetables with the highest glycemic index, such as potatoes,

beets, and carrots, have been labeled Funky Foods and eliminated altogether. Whole grains, beans, and dairy products have a moderate glycemic index and have been categorized in the Somersize Carbos group. And nonstarchy vegetables with the lowest glycemic index have been categorized in the Somersize Veggies group.

GLYCEMIC INDEX

Beer	110
Sugar	100
White bread	95
Instant potatoes	95
Honey	90
Jam	90
Cornflakes	85
Popcorn	85
Carrots	85
Potatoes	70
Pasta (from white flour)	65
Bananas	60
Dried fruit	60
Brown rice	50
Whole wheat bread	50
Whole wheat pasta	45
Fresh white beans	40
Oatmeal	40
Whole rye bread	40
Green peas	40
Whole cereals	35
Dairy products	35
Wild rice	35
Fresh fruits	35
Dried beans	30
Dark chocolate	22
Soy	15
Green vegetables	Less than 15

WHAT'S THE DEAL WITH DAIRY?

Many people, including me, get confused about dairy products with regard to Somersizing. When you're having a Pro/Fats meal, you may eat all the cheese you want and you may add cream to your sauce, but you can't use a splash of milk in your decaf coffee. When you're having a Carbos meal you can eat nonfat yogurt, but you can't use nonfat yogurt with a Pro/Fats meal. What's the deal? Let me help to clarify this issue.

Milk has protein and carbohydrates, whether it's nonfat, low-fat, or whole milk. Yogurt has protein and carbohydrates, whether it's nonfat, low-fat, or whole-milk yogurt. When we eat proteins or fats, we do not eat foods that contain carbohydrates; therefore, we cannot include any kind of milk or yogurt in the Pro/Fats meal. When we eat a Carbos meal, we can include products with protein, as long as they do not contain any fat. Therefore, we can include nonfat milk and nonfat yogurt. Low-fat and whole milk or yogurt are grouped as Funky Foods because they have fat and carbohydrates.

What about cream, butter, cheese, sour cream, and the like? These "milk" products have a very different quality than their plain milk or yogurt cousins. In the process of making cream, butter, or cheese, all the carbohydrates are processed out of these dairy products, leaving only the protein and fat. That is the reason why these dairy products without *carbohydrates are included in the Pro/Fats group, while the milk products with carbohydrates are grouped in the Carbos group.*

Get it? If not, read it again.

DAIRY PRODUCTS

PRO/FATS—DAIRY PRODUCTS WITHOUT CARBOHYDRATES	CARBOS—DAIRY PRODUCTS WITH CARBOHYDRATES AND NO FAT	FUNKY FOODS—DAIRY PRODUCTS WITH CARBOHYDRATES AND FAT
Butter	Nonfat milk	Low-fat milk
Cream	Nonfat yogurt	Whole milk
Cheese	Nonfat cheese	Low-fat yogurt
Sour cream	Nonfat soy milk	Whole-milk yogurt
Crème fraîche	Nonfat rice milk	Buttermilk
	Nonfat cottage cheese	Low-fat or whole soymilk
		Low-fat or whole rice milk

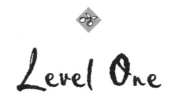

Level One

Now that you have a basic understanding of what foods to eliminate and how to categorize the rest of foods into our four Somersize Food Groups, you can get started on your new lifestyle. Let me walk you through each meal so you can see how easy it is to Somersize at every meal.

BREAKFAST

Each meal is an opportunity to eat something great, even on Level One when you're trying to lose weight. Let's talk about all the delicious breakfast options. I love breakfast! Cereal, toast, fruit, eggs, bacon, sausage . . . bring them on! As long as you follow the Somersize combinations, you may eat *any* of those foods for breakfast, just not in the same sitting. Here are your choices.

Breakfast #1—Fruit Meal
Breakfast #2— Carbos Meal
Breakfast #3— Fruit, wait twenty
   minutes, then Carbos Meal
Breakfast #4—Pro/Fats and Veggies Meal

Breakfast #1—Fruit Meal

Start your day off with a couple of plums, an orange, or half a cantaloupe. Or combine your favorite fruits in a blender with some juice and a few ice cubes for a frosty fruit smoothie. Or dice some mangoes, pineapple, papaya, and grapes for a tasty fruit salad. Remember, you may eat any kind of fruit, except bananas, which are a Funky Food. Fruit is best in the morning when eaten on an empty stomach. Fruit keeps you regular and is loaded with vitamins, nutrients, and a natural source of energy.

EXAMPLES OF BREAKFAST #1— FRUIT MEAL

- Fruit smoothie with peaches, raspberries, strawberries, and fruit juice
- Fruit smoothie with pineapple chunks, papaya, and orange juice
- Fruit salad of melon, grapes, and oranges
- An apple
- A bowl of fresh cherries
- A slice of watermelon

TO DRINK: Decaf coffee or tea—black (or sweetened with SomerSweet, or artificial sweetener if you must)

EXAMPLES OF BREAKFAST #2— CARBOS MEAL

- Whole wheat toast with nonfat cottage cheese and tomato
- Rye bagel with nonfat ricotta cheese
- Fat-free wheat tortilla with black beans and salsa
- Nonfat yogurt sprinkled with Grape Nuts
- Shredded wheat with nonfat milk
- Oatmeal with nonfat milk

TO DRINK: Decaf coffee or tea—black or with nonfat milk (and/or sweetened with SomerSweet, or artificial sweetener if you must)

Breakfast #2—Carbos Meal

Morning is the best time of the day to eat your Carbos so you can use the natural energy they supply throughout the day. There are a number of wonderful options to satisfy your hunger. I like whole-grain toast with nonfat cottage cheese or yogurt. Or I like hot or cold whole grain cereal with nonfat milk. Since we cannot combine any fat with our Carbos, this is the only time we choose fat-free products, specifically nonfat dairy products. I guard against choosing *processed* fat-free dairy products, like fat-free cream cheese, because they are often loaded with starches, fillers, and chemicals.

And remember, you may have Veggies with your Carbos, so feel free to top your toast with tomato and basil or a slice of red onion, if you like.

Breakfast #3— Fruit, wait twenty minutes, then Carbos Meal

Fruit, then Carbos is my favorite choice for breakfast because these foods provide me with necessary fiber and a whole host of vitamins and nutrients. Besides that, they just taste good! Alan is the master breakfast maker in our home. Usually he brings me a great fruit smoothie in the morning. Then I work out with my son-in-law, Frank, who is my personal trainer. Afterward we have toast or cereal with decaf coffee. Morning is the best time to eat your Fruit and Carbos so that you have plenty of time to burn off the natural sources of energy they provide.

Here are a few more examples of Fruit and Carbos.

- Melon. Wait twenty minutes.
  Oatmeal with nonfat milk and
  SomerSweet
- Fruit smoothie with cantaloupe,
  raspberries, and grapefruit juice.
  Wait twenty minutes.
  Whole-grain toast with nonfat cottage
  cheese and a sprinkle of cinnamon
- A couple of oranges. Wait twenty
  minutes.
  Puffed wheat cereal with nonfat milk
- Pineapple slices. Wait twenty minutes.
  Toasted rye bagel and a bowl of non-
  fat yogurt sweetened with a little
  vanilla extract
- Fruit salad. Wait twenty minutes.
- Cream of wheat with nonfat milk

TO DRINK: Decaf coffee or tea—black or
with nonfat milk (and/or sweetened with
SomerSweet, or artificial sweetener if you
must)

Breakfast #3—
Pro/Fats and Veggies Meal

In a Pro/Fats and Veggies breakfast, you may
have anything from the Pro/Fats group with
anything from the Veggies group. You have
so many choices with this breakfast. The
"incredible egg" can be scrambled, fried,
boiled, poached, or made into an omelette or
a frittata. Don't be afraid of the eggs! Have as
many as you like. Cook them up in butter or
oil and serve them with sausage or bacon (I
look for brands with no nitrates). Or try my
Mexican Omelette (p. 140). For additional

flavor, you can even cook your eggs in the
bacon fat or sausage fat. Some diet, huh? You
can have meat, fish, or poultry, including
chicken, shrimp, crab, lox, and smoked fish.
Feel free to add some cheese to that
omelette! And don't forget your Veggies, like
onions, tomatoes, zucchini, spinach, mushrooms, asparagus, and more. I have included
several egg dishes in the recipe section.

Here are just a few more examples of
what you might create for a Pro/Fats and
Veggies breakfast.

- Omelette—with zucchini, Swiss
  cheese, mushrooms, and sour cream
  Side of turkey sausage
- Fried eggs with bacon
  Side of tomatoes
- Scrambled eggs with smoked salmon,
  asparagus, and sour cream
- Huevos rancheros—fried eggs with
  caramelized onions, cheddar cheese,
  salsa, and sour cream
- Poached eggs on a bed of spinach with
  Canadian bacon and hollandaise sauce
  Side of green beans
- Fried eggs with ground chicken and
  spinach

TO DRINK: Decaf coffee or tea—black or
with cream (and/or sweetened with Somer-
Sweet, or artificial sweetener if you must)

Any of these foods would make up a perfectly combined Somersize breakfast, so you
may eat until you are full. This is a great
breakfast option when you're eating out
because there are so few restrictions. Just stay
away from toast, jelly, potatoes, and fruit
with your Pro/Fats and Veggies breakfast.

(If you want to start this meal with Fruit, you must wait one hour to have your Pro/Fats and Veggies.)

LUNCH AND DINNER

For lunch today, and every day, we are serving salads, soups, sandwiches, chicken, steak, fish, pasta, and more! You just have to decide what food group you feel like and then design a meal in the proper Somersize combination. Here are your choices.

Lunch or Dinner #1—
   Pro/Fats and Veggies Meal
Lunch or Dinner #2—
   Carbos and Veggies Meal
Lunch or Dinner #3—
   Single Food Group Meal

Lunch or Dinner #1— Pro/Fats and Veggies Meal

Flavor, flavor, flavor! That's what you can look forward to with every Pro/Fats and Veggies meal. Order from any restaurant menu with the Pro/Fats and Veggies Meal; meat, poultry, or fish can be grilled, broiled, baked, roasted, or fried and served with plenty of fresh vegetables, raw, steamed, sautéed, or grilled. Enjoy cooking with oil or butter and don't forget to add the cheese! Preparing meals for yourself at home or eating in a restaurant is a pleasure with the Pro/Fats and Veggies Meal. I have included many Pro/Fats and Veggies meals in the recipe section. Here are a few more examples.

EXAMPLES OF LUNCH OR DINNER #1—PRO/FATS AND VEGGIES MEAL

- Cobb salad with chicken, bacon, egg, tomato, blue cheese, and green onions with full-fat dressing of your choice. (Hold the avocado.)
- Taco salad with shredded beef, tomatoes, cheddar cheese, salsa, onions, and sour cream. (Hold the beans and chips.)
- Grilled fish with lemon butter sauce
  Snow peas tossed in butter
  Green salad with full-fat dressing of your choice
- Caesar salad (hold the croutons) with grilled chicken breast
  Grilled red peppers, zucchini, and fennel
- Hamburger patty with melted jack cheese and a pile of onions
  Green salad with cherry tomatoes and blue cheese dressing
- Egg salad tossed with celery, green onions, and mayonnaise served in lettuce cups with tomato slices and alfalfa sprouts
- Rotisserie style chicken
  Steamed broccoli and cauliflower covered with cheese
- Steamed crab legs and grilled filet mignon
  Steamed artichoke with butter or mayonnaise dip
  Butter lettuce salad with zucchini and Parmesan cheese
- Turkey cutlet served over sautéed Swiss chard with a butter wine sauce
  Green salad with goat cheese and candied tomatoes

- Grilled lamb chops with lemon and olive oil

  Greek salad with tomatoes, cucumber, red onion, feta cheese, and olive oil
- Stir-fried shrimp with napa cabbage, celery, broccoli, yellow peppers, Italian squash, bamboo shoots
- Chopped salad with salami, roasted peppers, tomatoes, onions, and provolone

  Fresh raw vegetables with dip
- Steak with peppercorn cream sauce and sautéed mushrooms

  Steamed green beans tossed in butter radicchio and endive salad with blue cheese and tomato

TO DRINK: Water, mineral water, decaf coffee or tea with cream (and/or sweetened with SomerSweet, or artificial sweetener if you must)

Your Pro/Fats and Veggies meals will range from the incredibly simple to the luxuriously extravagant. With so much to choose from you won't ever get bored eating the same old thing. In fact, your food will probably taste better than ever as you trim your way down to your ideal body weight.

Lunch or Dinner #2— Carbos and Veggies Meal

I choose this option very infrequently, because I prefer to eat my Carbos only in the morning when I'm trying to lose weight. But every now and then you just need a Carbo fix at lunch or dinner and it really hits the spot. You can have any whole grains or beans with nonfat dairy products and any of the vegetables in the Veggies list. Be careful when you look for *whole wheat products;* many manufacturers are now listing "wheat flour" for regular white flour because white flour starts from wheat. It must say *"whole* wheat flour" to really be a whole grain. In general, if it looks too white to be whole wheat . . . it probably is.

You might have brown rice with peas or black bean chili with fresh tomato salsa and whole wheat tortillas or whole grain pasta with tomato basil sauce or whole wheat pita bread with hummus, baba ganoush, and fresh vegetables. With any of these meals you could have a green salad. The key to the Carbos and Veggies Meal is to make sure there is absolutely no fat.

I have included a few Carbos and Veggies recipes in the recipe section. Here are more examples.

EXAMPLES OF LUNCH OR DINNER #2—CARBOS & VEGGIES MEAL

- Brown rice with soy sauce and steamed vegetables

  Green salad with a splash of vinegar
- Whole wheat pita bread with nonfat ricotta cheese, roasted peppers, and eggplant

  Grilled zucchini and yellow squash
- Whole wheat pasta with tomato, basil, and garlic sauce

  An artichoke with a squeeze of lemon
- A bowl of black beans with whole wheat tortillas and fresh salsa
- Whole wheat pita bread with hummus, baba ganoush, lettuce, and tomato

- Spinach whole wheat pasta with fresh garden vegetables, peas, and stewed tomatoes
- Whole wheat cheeseless pizza with marinara sauce, mushrooms, onions, tomatoes, and artichoke hearts
  Green salad with a squeeze of lemon.

TO DRINK: Water, mineral water, decaf coffee or tea with nonfat milk (and/or sweetened with SomerSweet, or artificial sweetener if you must)

This is a very satisfying and healthy option with all the whole grains and fresh vegetables. It can be a little restrictive, however, because on Level One you can't have any fat and you must watch for hidden sugars and Funky Foods. Because this meal is more difficult when you're eating in a restaurant, I normally prepare Carbos and Veggies at home.

Lunch or Dinner #3— Single Food Group Meal

Every now and then you might want to have a meal made up of only one food group, like the all Fruit meal or the all Veggies meal. Of course, this is perfectly fine on rare occasions, but I do not recommend it with any frequency.

FINDING A RHYTHM THAT WORKS

When I'm losing weight on Level One, I find that the fewer carbos I eat, the more results I see. As I explained earlier, carbos are an energy source and if you're not giving your body many sources of energy it will have to break down your fat reserves and use *them* as energy. But we don't want to cut out carbohydrates completely because they are an important source of fiber and help keep your system moving properly. And if you go too low with carbohydrates, your body will break down its protein, instead of its fat reserves, to be used as energy.

Here's what works best for me. I like to eat the Fruit, then Carbos breakfast. Because carbos are a good energy source, it's best to eat them in the morning so that you can use that energy throughout the day. For lunch or dinner I find more options with Pro/Fats and plenty of Veggies. Carbo meals for lunch and dinner are a little more restrictive because you can have absolutely no fat.

My recommendation is that for breakfast you have Breakfast #3—Fruit, then Carbos. For lunch and dinner I recommend Pro/Fats and Veggies as a rule with the Carbo and Veggies meal as the exception. If you eat too many carbohydrates, even the right kind of carbohydrates, they could get stored as fat for later use. (And if you're filling up on carbos, you're probably not giving your body enough protein and fat.) Remember, you're giving your body the small amount of carbohydrates it needs because your Pro/Fats and Veggies meals include some carbohydrates in the form of the many vegetables you'll be enjoying.

In fact, you could choose the Pro/Fats and Veggies meal at *every* meal and enjoy great health—it's a perfect combination of protein, fat, and carbohydrates (in the form of low-starch vegetables). (You know how I love my eggs with bacon or sausage in the morning!) This combination gives your body all the essential building materials it needs to thrive. The Carbos and Veggies meal gives you some diversity now and then and, as I said, includes all that great fiber.

This is only a blueprint of how I divide my Pro/Fats and Carbos meals. For me, those carbos tend to fatten me up like a corn-fed cow, especially at this age, when I am fighting even more hormonal imbalances. You may find, however, that your body can handle more carbohydrates and that you feel better eating mostly grains and vegetables. On the other hand, if you are eating mostly Pro/Fats, you must balance your meals with plenty of fresh vegetables. It is unwise to eat only meat and cheese without the fiber and nutrients added from vegetables.

YOU'RE ONLY CHEATING YOURSELF

My son, Bruce, has always had a beautiful, slim body. He wears a suit better than anyone I know (says the mother!). When he hit his thirties he started complaining of a "belly" for the first time in his life. I told him exactly what I tell you. "If you stand naked in front of the mirror and you are thick through the middle, then you have raised insulin levels. That means your cells are overloaded with sugar and will not accept any more. From that point on, any

sugar you eat, whether it's a candy bar or a carrot, will be stored as fat."

Bruce and his wife, Caroline, have been on Level Two for several years now, but Bruce decided to Somersize back on Level One until he got the problem under control. After living on Level One for a couple weeks, Bruce started complaining to Caroline that he was not losing the weight. She suggested they reexamine what he was eating to make sure he was following all of the Level One guidelines. Every day for breakfast he was eating a large bowl of cereal with nonfat milk. If the cereal is whole grain with no sugar, then this should not be a problem. When Caroline checked the ingredients she found that this "healthy" cereal Bruce had been eating for months was loaded with "cane juice," another name for sugar! In the back of his mind, Bruce knew it had sugar, but somehow he convinced himself it was okay.

Plus, he was drinking quite a bit of wine with dinner. When I thought about it, I realized that Bruce's minor weight gain coincided with his new hobby—wine. During the last two years, Bruce has started collecting fine wines. He's become quite the afficionado. For his birthday last year, Caroline threw him an intimate wine-tasting dinner at Spago, where Bruce served a horizontal tasting of ten of the finest wines from 1983. Wolfgang Puck cooked perhaps the most spectacular dinner I have ever eaten. He had just come home from Austria with the largest white truffle he had ever seen! He lavishly shaved the delicacy over our courses. French Bordeaux, fabulous food . . . it was divine.

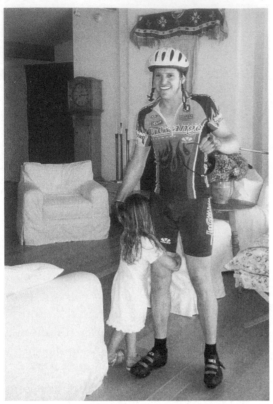

Bruce in full biking regalia.

When I asked Bruce how much wine he drinks he said about a glass or two every night. I told him he should cut back on the wine, because wine is received by the body as sugar. He groaned, but agreed. He made it very clear that he was Somersizing purely for vanity reasons—not for health reasons (though, of course, he'd be getting health benefits too)! As the mother, I was happy for him on both fronts.

Now Bruce is eating fruit in the morning. He waits an hour and then eats a big plate full of scrambled eggs with cheddar cheese and hot sauce. He's off the wine and he's become an avid cyclist. Plus, he's using

the Torso Track to target his abs! I am happy to report . . . my skinny boy is back on track, looking and feeling his best. He's slim and trim, which allows him to enjoy his wine again, but in greater moderation (like his mother).

I tell you Bruce's story because every now and then someone will tell me they are following all the Level One guidelines and they are still not losing weight. You cannot Somersize half heartedly on Level One. Reexamine your meals and make sure you are not sneaking in hidden sugars or Funky Foods. If you cheat, you are only cheating yourself. Cheating is for Level Two only.

Recently Alan and I hosted two of our dear friends for a weeklong vacation. Freddy is about sixty years old and is experiencing health problems. He's Type II diabetic and knows he needs to make a lifestyle change to turn his health around. Since Somersizing helps control insulin levels, Freddy was very interested in learning about it, so I cooked for him for an entire week and gave him a "hands-on" tutorial at meal after meal.

Freddy is a major bread addict. *He loves bread.* The hardest thing about Somersizing for him was giving up the bread. At our home I simply do not put it out, so he got by without it, but I knew how hard it was for him, evidenced by his frequent comments about how long it had been since he'd had bread. Like any other addictive substance, sugar and carbohydrates cause cravings, just like a drug addict craves the drug and the alcoholic craves the bottle. Sugar and white flour are addictive substances and Freddy has it bad!

One afternoon we went out for lunch and the waiter placed a basket of white rolls on the table. I saw my friend eyeing the bread. I hate being the food police, so I said to him, "Freddy, I am not your keeper. If you want the bread, don't worry about me. It's entirely up to you." We continued our conversation and before I knew it, Freddy had eaten three white flour rolls. He conceded, "Well, it's okay because at least I didn't have the butter." Then he went on to order a perfectly Somersized meal of chicken with butter sauce, salad, and sautéed vegetables.

He could have eaten as much butter as he wanted without any problem! It's the white flour that will raise his insulin level and cause the bread to be stored as fat—as well as rasing his blood sugar level, which is the problem of the Type II diabetic. And that lovely meal of chicken and butter sauce, which causes little to no insulin response, will now be trapped with the insulin from the bread.

YOU CANNOT SOMERSIZE HALFHEARTEDLY ON LEVEL ONE!

Without the presence of insulin, the amount of calories and fat grams you eat does not matter. This scenario changes drastically when you add foods that create the presence of insulin, such as sugar and carbohydrates. If you are eating foods that create an insulin response the entire mass of food has the potential to be stored as fat. Now the calories and fat grams *do* matter because

there's simply more energy to be converted to fat.

If you are going to cheat, cheat with an isolated food rather than adding it to a large meal. For instance, if Freddy really wanted bread, he should have eaten it alone, or better yet, with a salad. The fiber in salad helps diminish the effects of the insulin. Plus, salad is low in calories and fat, so at least if you're going to send a meal to the fat reserves, it is only bread and salad. You can eat the chicken with butter sauce, vegetables, and full-fat salad dressing without a problem, but if you add the bread you now put a high-fat and high-calorie meal at risk of being converted to fat. Stay on Level One until you feel the full effects. When your cells are unloaded from the built-up sugar, you can eat some sugars and carbs in moderation.

The moral of the story is . . . if you are not seeing results, you are probably cheating without even knowing it. Reexamine your meals, then reread all the food lists to make sure you are on track. If you are doing everything right and still not seeing results, consider cutting down on the amount of Fruit and Carbos meals you are eating. If you still do not see results, you may have a hormonal imbalance that requires hormone replacement therapy. (See Chapter 7 for more information.)

When you graduate to Level Two, your body will be able to handle a small amount of insulin because you have created room in your cells to store the small amount of sugar. Don't get cocky and overdo it! If you cheat too much, like Bruce, your cells will fill up with sugar and you'll have to go back to Level One until you correct the problem.

WHAT DO YOU MEAN, CHEAT? NOW WE HAVE SOMERSWEET!

I have always said, when you first start Somersizing, make sure you stick to the Level One guidelines while your body is unloading all the stored sugar from your cells. Creating imbalances, especially in the beginning, will spike your insulin levels and reverse all your hard work. It can be hard at first, so in the past I included some recipes with saccharin that would give you a sweet fix, but I told you to eat them only occasionally because of the harmful chemicals in artificial sweeteners. Now I have discovered the sweet and natural solution, Somer-Sweet!

I am so excited about this miracle sweetener! Now you can eat ice cream and cheesecake and chocolate mousse on Level One, guilt-free! SomerSweet is a natural, sweet fiber that won't spike your insulin levels and it's 99.9% chemical free! It's made from a special blend of fiber, fructose, and soy. It's sugar free and has less than 1 gram of carbohydrate per serving! That means you can enjoy it with all the food groups!

You'll feel like you're cheating when you enjoy the clean taste of SomerSweet stirred into your coffee or tea. You'll feel like a kid again when you sprinkle it on your morning cereal. You'll feel like you've died and gone to heaven when you eat rich and sinful desserts! With SomerSweet, now you can Eat, *Cheat*, and Melt the Fat Away! It's a miracle.

In the recipe section, you will see several Level One desserts made with SomerSweet. My Vanilla Bean Ice Cream is to die for! Ice cream is usually made with cream and milk, but since milk has carbohydrates, I make mine with all cream. Now that we have SomerSweet, you can dive into a bowl of pure vanilla ice cream with no sugar and no chemicals. It's so rich and creamy, you won't believe it! In fact, it's so rich, I serve it in small bowls because a little bit really fills you up. Remember, since it's made with all Pro/Fats, you may eat it after any Pro/Fats meal.

I have also included several recipes that I call *"Almost* Level One" desserts. These recipes are very close to Level One, with only a small amount of carbohydrates, usually from the addition of unsweetened cocoa powder. Now that we have SomerSweet, I can give you chocolaty desserts without any sugar or chemicals. Chocolate Truffles with no sugar! Dark Chocolate Ice Cream with no sugar! Molten Chocolate Cakes with no sugar! Fudgysicles on a stick with no sugar! The only imbalance comes from the cocoa powder, which is still considered a Funky Food because it contains caffeine and small amounts of carbohydrates. When you first begin Somersizing, I would recommend you stick to the Level One desserts. Let your body get to the point where The Melt begins and you see that fat start melting off your body. Once you are losing weight steadily, try incorporating these "Almost Level One" desserts. I doubt your weight loss will be disrupted, but you can test it for yourself.

This introduction of SomerSweet makes me so happy for all of us! It's hard to give up the taste of sugar, but the benefits are essential to our health and well-being. Millions have turned to artificial sweeteners, which contain harmful chemicals and side effects. Now we truly can enjoy the sweet treats we love with all-natural SomerSweet. Go ahead, my fellow Somersizers. Eat, *Cheat*, and Melt the Fat Away!

A SAMPLE WEEK ON LEVEL ONE

Even after all the explanation and all the recipes, people still ask me, "Well, what do *you* eat?" I tell them that I may have a Carbos breakfast and then a Pro/Fats and Veggies lunch . . . and they say, "No, I mean literally, what did you eat today for every meal and every snack? And what did you eat yesterday and the day before that?"

To tell you the truth, I don't think about every meal with such detail because this way of eating has become second nature to me. In an effort to give you an example of all the ways you can eat, I have written down absolutely everything I ate for an entire week so you could have an example of a whole week's worth of meals on Level One. I have not included portion size because, as you know, you simply eat until you are full. Your own meals can vary from mine tremendously, but perhaps this will give you some additional ideas for meal plans. (Many of these recipes can be found in this book, or in *Eat Great, Lose Weight* and *Get Skinny on Fabulous Food*.)

SUNDAY

9:00 Breakfast
   Spinach-Parmesan Frittata (p. 138)
   Side of turkey sausage
   Decaf coffee

1:00 Lunch at Home
   Tuna salad with celery, onions, and
      mayo served in lettuce cups

4:00 Snack on the Beach
   Two peaches

7:00 Family Dinner
   Beef Stew (p. 242) with onions, celery,
      mushrooms, and green beans
   Green salad with vinaigrette

MONDAY

Breakfast
   (7:00) Fruit smoothie (peaches,
      raspberries, orange juice)
   (7:30) Whole wheat toast with nonfat
      cottage cheese
   Decaf coffee

10:00 Snack
   Apple

1:00 Lunch
   Grilled Ginger Shrimp on Skewers
      (p. 213) as an appetizer
   Caesar Salad (p. 173) with grilled
      chicken (no croutons)

4:00 Snack
   A hard-boiled egg

7:30 Dinner
   Pork Chops with Creamy Shallot Sauce
      (p. 228)
   Steamed asparagus
   Salad with red leaf lettuce, tomatoes,
      fresh mozzarella, basil, and balsamic
      vinaigrette

TUESDAY

7:00 Breakfast
Fried eggs with crisp bacon

1:00 Lunch
Southern Country Fried Chicken Salad
(p. 178)

7:00 Dinner
Florentine Steak (p. 247)
Steamed broccoli and cauliflower with
lemon garlic butter
Butter lettuce salad with garlic
vinaigrette

9:00 Snack
A plum

WEDNESDAY

Breakfast
(6:00) Honeydew melon
(6:45) Decaf cappuccino with nonfat
milk
(9:00) Toasted pumpernickel bagel
Nonfat yogurt

2:00 Lunch
Baby greens with Parmesan cheese,
sun-dried tomatoes, and chicken
breast

6:00 Dinner at a Restaurant
Flattened Chicken (p. 222)
Assorted grilled vegetables
Radicchio, arugula, endive salad with
Parmesan cheese

9:00 Snack
A piece of cheddar cheese

THURSDAY

7:00 Breakfast
Scrambled eggs with turkey sausage links
Decaf coffee

10:00 Snack
Piece of string cheese

1:00 Lunch
Taco salad—romaine lettuce, ground
beef, cheddar cheese, salsa, sour
cream, salsa (no beans, tortillas, or
guacamole)

4:00 Snack
Whole wheat pretzels (no-fat)

7:30 Dinner
Pan-Fried Petrale Sole with Lemon,
Butter, and Caper Sauce (p. 216)
Steamed artichoke with lemon dill
mayonnaise

9:30 Dessert
Vanilla Bean Ice Cream (p. 250)

FRIDAY

Breakfast
(9:00) Papaya
(9:30) Shredded wheat with nonfat milk

12:30 Lunch
Cobb salad—lettuce, blue cheese,
turkey, bacon, tomato, green onion,
hard-boiled egg, blue cheese dressing
(no avocado)

3:00 Snack
An orange

6:00 Dinner
Green salad with blue cheese and
balsamic vinaigrette
Chicken Cacciatore (chicken, tomato,
peppers, onions, olive oil, garlic)
Sugarless Fudgysicle (p. 252)

SATURDAY

9:00 Breakfast
Mangoes and strawberries

Decaf nonfat cappuccino

1:00 Lunch
Middle Eastern Vegetable Stew (p. 206)
Vegetable sticks with hummus

6:30 Dinner
Baby Lamb Chops with Parmesan
Crusts and Sweet Tomato Sauce
(p. 234)
Grilled zucchini and eggplant
Green salad with Brie and red wine
vinaigrette

8:30 Dessert
Tangerines

SOMERSIZING TIPS

I realize this program may seem a bit overwhelming at first, but soon you will discover how simple Somersizing can be. Whenever my friends and family first start the program, they frequently call me with questions. And since I can't give my home phone number to everyone, I have compiled some helpful tips for dining out and eating at home.

Tips for Dining Out

So many people tell me, "I eat two to three meals each day in restaurants; it's impossible to lose weight." Once you understand Somersizing, eating in any restaurant is truly easy. First I scan the menu and decide if I want to choose a Pro/Fats and Veggies meal or a Carbos and Veggies meal. Ninety-five percent of the time I'll choose a Pro/Fats meal, which might be a green salad with dressing of my choice, a chicken, meat, or fish entree with a lovely sauce, and plenty of steamed, sauteed, or grilled vegetables. On the rare occasion that I choose to have a Carbos and Veggies meal, I might order a vegetarian sandwich on whole-grain bread or brown rice with steamed vegetables and soy sauce.

The key to the Pro/Fats meal is no bread, pasta, potatoes, or rice. We are accustomed to beginning every meal in a restaurant by emptying a basket of bread into our bellies before we even order! Then we eat a meal of meat with potatoes or a turkey sandwich or a Chinese chicken salad piled high with fried rice noodles and wontons. Add a couple of glasses of caffeine, like iced tea or diet

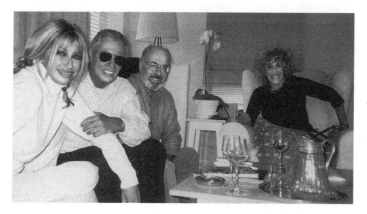

Alan and me with our dear friends Arthur and Susie (Susie is the best cook I know).

cola, and you have a recipe for metabolic disaster. These are the things that throw your system into chaos.

You'll be surprised at how quickly you'll get over missing the starch. Make sure to watch for hidden sugars or starches in the salad dressings or sauces. Drill your server a little to get the information you need; ask the kitchen to substitute extra vegetables or salad for the starchy side dish. Just make sure all the vegetables are on the Veggies list. It does you no good to get a big side dish of sautéed carrots. And it's a terrible waste of food to be served items you know you cannot eat.

You will also have to get over that feeling of being "overstuffed" when you finish a meal. I used to think I was not full until my stomach became distended and I could not consider putting another bite into my mouth. When you Somersize you will not get that overstuffed feeling, because your body is not fighting with bad food combinations that cause digestive problems. Your system becomes cleansed and you become accustomed to feeling satisfied without feeling stuffed.

The Level One Carbos meal is much more restrictive when you're eating out. It must be fat free so that all those carbohydrates are burned off rather than stored as fat. Also, watch out for sugars and hidden Funky Foods, and avoid anything from the Pro/Fats group; meat and cheese on that sandwich would throw your system into a tizzy. Even mayonnaise, oil, and avocado are not okay on Level One with carbos.

With minimal effort, you can enjoy any restaurant and still lose weight. And it's worth it! Try and judge for yourself. I guarantee you'll like the way you feel when you Somersize. No bloating or gas, improved elimination, and more energy than ever before.

Tips for Eating at Home

As far as eating at home, if you're used to eating prepared foods, you will need to make some adjustments. Most prepared foods are made with processed products like sugar, white flour, and a variety of unpronounceable chemicals. Say good-bye to Hamburger Helper! With a little preparation, you can learn to create fresh foods that taste much better and are far more nutritious. I keep my refrigerator stocked with ingredients that allow me to prepare meals quickly. I like to shop at our local farmer's market on Saturdays and stock up for the week. Alan and I make a morning of it. We each grab a couple of straw bags and scan the market for the selections of the season. Alan heads straight for the fruit growers—succulent melons, crisp apples, peaches, berries, pomegranates, whatever the season brings. I gravitate toward the vegetable stands. My friend at the mushroom stand will put together a brown bag with his prized shiitake and oyster mushrooms. The lettuce growers display a variety of romaine, endive, radicchio, frisée, baby spinach, butter lettuce, and more. I pick up a bag of sugar snap peas, broccoli, cauliflower, green beans, asparagus, onions, leeks, and vine-ripened tomatoes—all grown organically without pesticides.

On Sundays I do a little cooking; perhaps I'll make some mushroom-sausage stuffing with my shiitakes and stuff a small turkey. The next day I'll use the leftover meat for turkey salad served in lettuce cups, and then I'll take the carcass and make a delicious turkey and vegetable soup for the following night.

Having ingredients in the house makes coming home from work and preparing dinner so easy. Most of the recipes in this book are quick and require minimal skills as a chef. The most important part of any good recipe is finding good, quality ingredients. You'll find when you shop

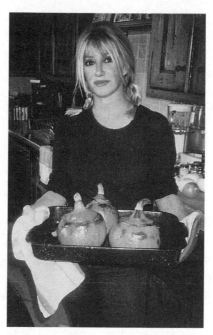

Yum! Baked Pumpkins.

that you'll mostly buy foods from the perimeter of the grocery store. Start in the produce section for all your fresh fruits and vegetables. Then the meat and fish section. Try to look for a great butcher who sells meat without added hormones, nitrates, or preservatives. Go to the bakery to look for fresh bread or bagels made from whole grains. And then stock up in the dairy department on butter, sour cream, cheese, nonfat milk and yogurt. I always feel good at the checkout stand when I unload my groceries because I'll have several wrapped packages from the butcher, a ton of bags from the produce section, and a great selection of cheeses and dairy products. There are no boxes of cookies, crackers, or snack food. It's all *real* food, as close to its natural state as possible.

I get so many letters from people saying they have a hard time finding ingredients for my recipes. Feel free to substitute! I use whatever's available, and I invite you to do the same. If you cannot find arugula, use another green leafy vegetable like spinach, dandelion, or mustard greens. Also, check out specialty shops like Dean & Deluca. They have a mail order catalog (1-877-826-9246) and a Web site (www.deandeluca.com).

To give you an idea of what I shop for each week, I've listed some of the ingredients I always like to have in my refrigerator and pantry.

Whole-grain bread: Whole wheat, pumpernickel, rye; whatever kind you like. Keep an extra loaf in the freezer so you never run out. Check for hidden sugars, fats, fruits, or sweeteners. Choose totally natural breads made without honey or white flour or fruit juice. I have found Ezekial (made from sprouted grain). Again, make sure you look for *whole* wheat, not just *wheat flour*. Many manufacturers are listing white flour now as wheat flour to make you think it is a healthier product. Don't be fooled. White flour begins with a grain of wheat . . . it just gets processed so extensively that none of the nutrients of the original wheat remain in the end product. Sometimes it's difficult to find bread that fits all these requirements. Ask your local bakery if they make all whole wheat bread. Flatbreads are excellent choices and readily available—whole wheat pita, whole wheat lavash bread, and whole wheat tortillas. Just make sure they're made without any fats.

Whole-grain pastas: Some whole wheat pastas can be mushy, so you may have to try out a few. I like De Cecco brand whole wheat best. Whatever brand you choose, look for whole wheat or durum whole wheat semolina. I also like whole wheat and artichoke pasta. Straight semolina on its own is not allowed. Also try pastas made from whole grains like kamut, spelt, or brown rice.

Hot cereals: Oatmeal and Cream of Wheat.

Cold cereals: I like Shredded Wheat, Grape Nuts, Puffed Wheat, and Crispy Brown Rice. Again, check for sugars and Funky Foods carefully on the labels.

Nonfat cottage cheese: Great on your toast in the morning or for a snack in the afternoon.

Nonfat yogurt: A good-quality plain nonfat yogurt is a delicious treat. Pavel's is my favorite brand, but it's sometimes hard to find.

Nonfat milk: I buy the kind from farms that don't use any hormones, pesticides, or antibiotics.

Beans: Dried, canned, or fresh. I like cannelini beans, pinto beans, lentils, black-eyed peas, and garbanzo beans (also called chickpeas).

Mustard: Yellow, whole-grain, and Dijon.

Rice: Brown rice and wild rice. Make sure neither is blended with white rice of any sort.

Phyllo dough: Many types are whole wheat. Keep a box in the freezer for quick Level Two tarts and pastries.

Cheese: Whatever kind you like. I always have buffalo mozzarella and goat cheese in the fridge. I also try to keep Stilton or another good blue, Romano, and feta on hand. My favorite Parmesan is Parmiggiano-Reggiano. Pecorino is wonderful and sometimes I splurge on a triple cream like Camembert or Brie. On most diets celery is the only free food that can be eaten at will. Who knew cheese could keep you so lean and healthy! Keep little individually wrapped cheeses, like string cheese or Laughing Cow, on hand for snacks.

Butter: There's nothing like the real flavor of butter. I keep salted and sweet on hand.

Fresh eggs: I get mine from the farmer's market for the freshest of fresh. I like to keep some hard-boiled in the fridge for quick snacks.

Mayonnaise: Best Foods or Hellman's is my favorite brand. I used to avoid it in Level

One because it has sugar listed in the ingredients. But if you look on the label you'll notice there are zero carbohydrates per serving. I presume the added sugar must be in trace amounts or there would be an increased carbohydrate listing. So enjoy your Best Foods. Or make your own with my easy recipe.

Fresh seafood: I always buy my seafood the same day I eat it. My favorites are sea bass, trout, tuna, shrimp, and scallops. The exception to the freshness rule are frozen Alaskan king crab legs, and shrimp. They're expensive, but an amazing treat and a cinch to make.

Meat: I like to keep a few things in the freezer to thaw for a quick meal. Pork chops, lean ground beef, steaks, and lamb chops. Remember, the fat in meat is *real* fat, which promotes healthy cells.

Oil: I buy extra virgin olive oil by the case. I use it in almost every meal. I also keep vegetable oil, like safflower or canola. And don't forget hot chili oil and sesame oil to flavor those delicious Asian meals.

Vinegar: Balsamic, red wine, white wine, and champagne vinegar are my household staples. Rice vinegar is good to have around for Asian dishes.

Poultry: I eat a lot of chicken. I have the butcher make a few packages with two chicken breasts in each. That way I can keep them in the freezer and thaw them quickly for an easy meal. Same with turkey cut-lets—they're a nice alternative with a slightly different flavor. I also keep ground chicken and ground turkey on hand.

Lettuce: I buy my lettuce on the weekend and completely wash, dry, and bag it so that I have easy salads all week long (or buy pre-washed lettuce). I like red leaf, butter lettuce, romaine, radicchio, and endive.

Onions: Brown, red, scallions, and leeks. You'll see from my recipes, I can make any meal great by starting with onions!

Garlic: And plenty of it. Sometimes I peel a couple heads and keep the cloves in olive oil in the fridge for quick access.

Ginger: Fresh and ground for Asian recipes.

Soy sauce: For Asian recipes.

Fresh veggies: Whatever is in season and looks great—asparagus, broccoli, cauliflower, tomatoes, summer squash, zucchini, fennel, celery, celery root, green beans, bell peppers, etc. You'll be eating a lot of vegetables to make up for the missing starch, so load up.

Canned goods: I always keep canned tomatoes on hand for easy-to-prepare sauces. I buy tomato sauce, crushed tomatoes, and whole peeled tomatoes. I also like hearts of palm, which are great in salads. Canned bamboo shoots are good for Asian dishes, and a couple cans of tuna fish are nice to have around to throw into salads. And I always keep cans of chicken and beef stock on hand for the times when I can't make my own. Watch for hidden sugars or starches. Hain is my favorite brand because it has no preservatives and it tastes great.

Frozen vegetables: I only use frozen vegetables when I absolutely can't get them fresh. The flavor doesn't compare.

Fresh and dried herbs: Basil, thyme, rosemary, parsley, tarragon, dill, mint, and cilantro are a few that I always like to have around. Most of these are easy to grow yourself if you have a sunny spot.

Fresh fruits: I choose whatever is in season—apples, grapes, mangoes, papaya, melons, berries, citrus fruits, and more. Remember, because their sugar content is so low, lemons and limes can be used to season foods from any of the four Somersize Food Groups.

Frozen fruits: Great for fruit smoothies and Level Two pastries. I always have frozen berries, peaches, pineapple, papaya, and mango when I can find them.

What to Drink?

Water. I highly recommend you drink eight to ten glasses of water a day. But try not to drink *with* your meals, because water can dilute your digestive juices, which slows down the digestive process. Your stomach acids are strongest right before you begin a new meal. When you eat, the acids break down the food quickly and pass it from the stomach. If you drink a big glass of water before your meal, these gastric juices become diluted and are less effective at breaking down the food. Therefore, if you must drink with your meal, eat a portion of your food before you drink anything so as not to dilute the strength of the gastric juices. It's best to drink your eight to ten glasses between meals. Besides water, you can also have decaffeinated coffee, teas, and even diet sodas, if you must. Personally, you already know why I stay away from soft drinks: they are loaded with dangerous chemicals. You would be doing your body a favor to eliminate them as well.

Don't Skip Meals

Whether you're eating at home or dining in restaurants, make sure not to skip meals. Our mothers always told us that breakfast is the most important meal of the day, right? In many ways they were correct. Your body has been fasting while you sleep, so when you wake up in the morning you have gone for some eight or ten hours without food. If you skip breakfast and don't eat until lunch, your body has gone twelve to fourteen hours without food. When you finally eat lunch, your body's survival instinct kicks in. It doesn't know when you're going to feed it again, so it hangs on to every morsel instead of properly processing the food. Remember to eat at least three meals a day—or eat more smaller meals throughout the day if you prefer.

Portion Control

People often ask me about portion size because they are used to feeling deprived on diets. Somersizing does not require you to measure any of your foods. You simply eat until you are full. At first you may need to eat more food to feel satisfied because you are accustomed to having that "stuffed" feeling when you finish a meal. You will not feel "stuffed" or bloated when you eat in proper combinations. I don't worry about you eating *too* much because it is difficult to overeat when you are eating only nutritious foods because your body will signal you when it is satiated. Overeating junk food, however, is a cinch because you can eat and eat and eat without ever giving your body what it needs to thrive! Your body may keep sending hunger messages until you give it the nutritious food it craves.

Get Moving

Exercise is an important part of any weight loss program. That doesn't mean you have to spend three hours a day in aerobics class. I realize that not everyone has the time or the money to join a gym and work out every day. I know with my busy schedule that it's hard to find the time to exercise

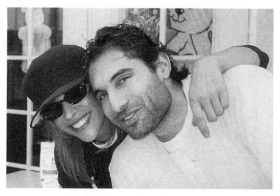

My stepdaughter, Leslie, and her husband, Frank.

regularly. When I'm home I try to work out as much as I can with my son-in-law, Frank Buffa. My stepdaughter, Leslie, has been married to Frank for five years. He is the former Mr. France and the best personal trainer I've ever worked with. I especially like our workouts when he brings our darling granddaughter Daisy along.

Frank comes to our house in the morning and takes Alan and me through a workout of resistance training. What a difference it has made in my muscle tone! Just thirty minutes a day, three times a week (except when I travel). Thanks to my Torso Track and my ThighMaster, my arms are no longer floppy, my tummy is tightening, my thighs are firm, and my backside is moving on up!

Somersizing helps me stay at the right weight. Exercising helps me keep the right shape. And it makes you feel great! Just make sure that you're giving your body the protein and fat it needs to build muscle while you're exercising. A low-fat, high-carbohydrate diet in combination with strenuous exercise is a recipe for disaster. Your muscles and bones can deteriorate without the proper nutrients to keep them healthy and strong.

Get yourself out and start moving. My motto is "Be fit, not fanatic." On the days when you just cannot find time for a workout, take a walk, just a twenty-minute walk, in the morning or the afternoon. Play tag with your kids. Take the stairs instead of the elevator. Take an active look at your activity level. Exercise helps you build lean muscle mass, which is a key element in losing weight. Lean muscle mass helps you burn calories twenty-four hours a day.

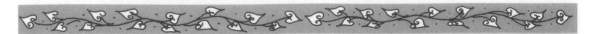

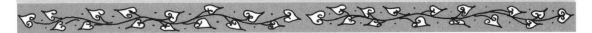

Plus, exercise is another way to keep insulin levels balanced. It helps us release the stored sugar from our cells so that we can get down to burning our fat reserves and losing that extra weight. So get out there and get moving. Find an activity that brings you enjoyment—it doesn't have to cost money—it just has to get you breathing a little harder.

Be Diligent!

As long as you are following *all* the Level One guidelines, you may eat until you are full and still lose weight. Be diligent! You cannot Somersize half heartedly. Your body is in the process of healing as it unloads years of stored away sugar in its cells. In order to retrain your body to burn your fat reserves, you must not confuse it by slipping up with bad combinations or Funky Foods. Besides, you have so many choices, there is no need to slip up. You will love eating this way and seeing the amazing results. Some people see results immediately and lose 5 or more pounds in the first week. Others don't see results until the second, third, or even fourth week. Be patient! You body is detoxifying from all the sugar and chemicals and bad combinations to which it has become accustomed. You *will* see results and once it begins you'll start to melt away down to your ideal body weight. Best of all, you'll love eating this way!

I have synthesized all the information you need to know for Level One in the Reference Guide, which you'll find in the back of the book. Use this guide as a reminder of which foods belong in what categories. In no time, you will get the hang of Somersizing and it will all become second nature.

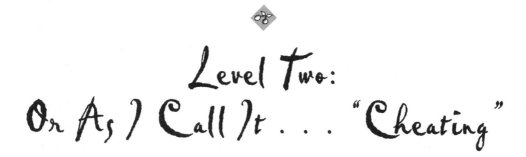

TWELVE

Level Two: Or As I Call It . . . "Cheating"

When you stand naked in front of the mirror and you are thin through the middle, and you are feeling happy with the way you are looking, you can graduate to Level Two, which is the maintenance portion of Somersizing. Level Two is simply Level One with cheating. Look, we are human beings, and every once in a while that scrumptious dessert the restaurant is offering looks too good to pass up. Your insulin levels are balanced, which is evident from your beautiful new slim waistline, so you can afford to indulge every once in a while.

Everyone cheats in different ways. I find I rarely create an imbalance cheating on sugary desserts. The sugars I miss the most are a glass of wine once or twice a week. Wine is accepted by the body as sugar. When I drink a glass of wine or two, I know I have created a slight imbalance. As a result I will go back to Level One for the next two or three meals. You have to be the judge as to

how many times a week you can cheat. When your pants are feeling tight, or your waistband starts cutting into your skin, it is time to go back to Level One. I used to be able to cheat more without having any adverse effects on my body. Now I find that if I keep my cheating to a couple of times a week, I can maintain my figure. That means two glasses of wine, and one scrumptious dessert. If I cheat any more than that, I find I start getting thick through the middle.

It's comforting to know that there are no foods that are forbidden. Somersizing simply asks that you first lose the unwanted weight, and when you have reached your goal, you can begin to incorporate the sugars you miss the most, in moderation. That is called cheating. You are your own policeman. You can't blow it. If you find that you have gotten off the Somersizing track, simply go back to Level One and resume eating delicious, flavorful foods, but be sure to eliminate all sugars, so you can give your body a chance to lower its insulin levels, and metabolize the foods you are ingesting efficiently.

In general, I live on Level One for the most part. Level Two involves cheating to some degree or another, so I remain vigilant because I do not want to go back to struggling with my weight. I am in control of my weight by Somersizing. I have been eating this way for ten years. The reason I know I will eat this way for the rest of my life is that Somersizing recognizes how human we all are. If you are craving or missing certain foods, have them, and then return to Level One eating.

But don't slip back into bad habits. In Level One you have trained your pancreas not to oversecrete insulin by eliminating Funky Foods. And rather than fill up on empty carbohydrates that give your body a quick source of energy, you have trained your body to use your fat reserves as an energy source. You've conditioned your system to digest quickly and efficiently by cutting out bad combinations. You have released the stored sugar from your cells and healed your metabolism. Now your body is in great shape and can handle a few imbalances.

The last thing we want is for all your hard work to be thrown away by resuming old habits. Level Two is about helping you find a balance so you can enjoy previously forbidden foods in moderation, without completely throwing caution to the wind. In Level Two, *you* are the only person who can determine how much imbalance your body can handle. Some people have to stay very close to Level One guidelines, with a minor

imbalance here and there, in order to maintain their weight. Other people find they can create quite a few imbalances and still maintain their weight. By using trial and error on your own body, you will soon know how many imbalances your body can handle. I know I've created too much of an imbalance when I feel bloated after a meal. Another warning sign for me is if I feel tired an hour or two after a meal. These are signs that I have wavered too far from Level One and need to pull in the reins. Of course, the most obvious sign is if you start to gain weight. Then you know you need to cut back on the treats and get back to eating cheese!

There are specific guidelines necessary to lose weight in Level One, and if you've gotten down to your goal weight, you have followed them diligently. I wish I could give you specific guidelines for Level Two, but actually that's the beauty of it . . . there are no hard-and-fast rules for Level Two. You are in control of your body and you need to find a rhythm you can live with for the rest of your life.

The great thing is that no matter how large an imbalance you create, you can always find your equilibrium. Level Two is really an extension of Level One, with a few indulgences here and there. Of course, moderation is the key to maintaining your weight. I find that if I eat a Level One lunch, like a Cobb salad with chicken, cheese, bacon, green onions, and tomatoes, every now and then I can add a piece of whole-grain bread without upsetting my system too much. Or if I wanted to indulge myself a little more, I would hold the bread and maybe have a piece of flourless chocolate cake. Certainly I would not have chocolate cake every day or it would catch up with me. And I would not eat the Cobb salad with the wheat bread *and* the cake, because that would be more carbohydrates than I could handle. Of course, a Cobb salad with a *white*-flour roll and the cake would mean bloat city.

I also find that on Level Two I can handle a few more Carbos and Veggies meals, but it seems the older I get, the fewer carbohydrates my body can handle. Whereas in Level One I eat my carbos almost exclusively at breakfast, on Level Two I might incorporate an occasional lunch and dinner revolving around whole wheat pasta or brown rice. Again, only you can determine how many of these Carbos meals you can eat without upsetting your system.

MIXING PRO/FATS AND CARBOS

As your system becomes clean you will find that your body can handle a small amount of carbohydrate *with* your Pro/Fats meals. When you combine carbohydrate with Pro/Fats, stay within the Carbos list. For instance, you might add one slice of buttered whole wheat toast with your eggs in the morning, but a stack of pancakes made from white flour would be overdoing it. Or you could have a tuna melt on one slice of whole-grain bread for lunch, but the side of potato salad would not be advised. For dinner you might have a small portion of wild rice with your chicken and vegetables, but

a side of white pasta would be too much.

Every now and then you may really want those pancakes or potato salad or pasta. Just make sure the imbalance is really worth it to you. Then go back and eat a few strict Level One meals for a while until you get your system back in balance. That's how Level Two works; you eat mostly on Level One and decide when you want to treat yourself. Sometimes I stay close to Level One with frequent, but small little treats here and there, like a little olive oil on my pasta or some wild rice in my chicken soup. Other times I stay strictly on Level One for a series of meals and then have a big treat (once a month), like a piece of birthday cake with buttercream frosting.

Every once in a while Alan and I like to eat Cheerios. They have a small amount of sugar, and I generally find I can eat Cheerios in the morning (on Level Two) without upsetting my system too much. However, the other night, we really went overboard. It was the end of March, which is an exciting time when you live in Los Angeles, because it's Oscar time. This year Alan and I were invited to the Vanity Fair party. It was quite an extravaganza! There were so many huge celebrities, it was a fascinating night to mingle and chat with everyone. One of the best parts was seeing all the fabulous gowns and jewels. I loved my dress. It was a creation by my incredibly talented stepdaughter, the designer Leslie Hamel.

When we wrapped up our night, at about two in the morning, Alan and I made our way home in the limousine. Like a child at the end of a day at Disneyland, Alan fell asleep within two minutes. By the time we got home and crawled into bed, it was after three o'clock in the morning. Unfortunately, I had to work very early the next morning, so the alarm went off at five. We managed to make our way through the day, but were exhausted from our long night of parties.

What does all of this have to do with Cheerios, you say? When we returned home that evening, we were so tired I could not bear the thought of making dinner. In fact, I was so tired I couldn't even pick up the phone and order out. So you know what we ate for dinner? Cheerios. We crawled into bed with two bowls, a half gallon of milk, and a box of Cheerios! Then we took all those carbs and went right to sleep.

Although I certainly don't recommend a box of Cheerios at dinner, on Level Two you have the freedom to blow it and then get right back on track. So we ate Cheerios for dinner. I didn't explode. I just got right back on track and started the next day with good old bacon and eggs.

Caroline and Bruce had a similar experience. They own a production company and were off for the day shooting a Visa commercial. It was a long day so they didn't get to eat dinner with the kids like they normally do. When they got home, they gave the girls a bath and put them to bed. By the time the kids were sleeping, it was past nine o'clock and Caroline just didn't feel like eating dinner. Bruce threw a salad together for himself, but Caroline decided to blow it and eat popcorn for dinner. She popped a bag of popcorn and crawled in bed. After eating about half of it, she wrapped the

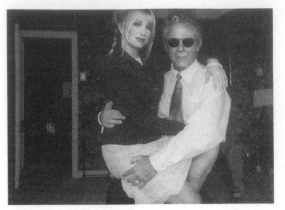

Alan and me in Paris going to the Samel L'Amboise for dinner.

popcorn in a dish towel and placed it on the floor next to her bed.

At three in the morning, she woke up to the sound of the crinkling popcorn bag! Quickly she woke Bruce up and said, "I think there's something in my popcorn bag!" When she looked over the edge of the bed, she saw the shadow of a mouse scampering away! Bruce turned on the flashlight and after giving the bag a few pokes, he removed it to the kitchen trash. Caroline said she will never eat popcorn for dinner again!

Generally I find that on Level Two I can eat a few more Carbos meals without a problem and I can add a little bit of fat. Sometimes I have whole-grain pasta or brown rice for lunch with vegetables. On Level One I have no oil with this meal, but on Level Two I can sauté the vegetables in some oil and have a more flavorful stir-fry without causing a significant imbalance. But adding protein to a Carbos meal is a little tricky. If I want to have meat with my pasta

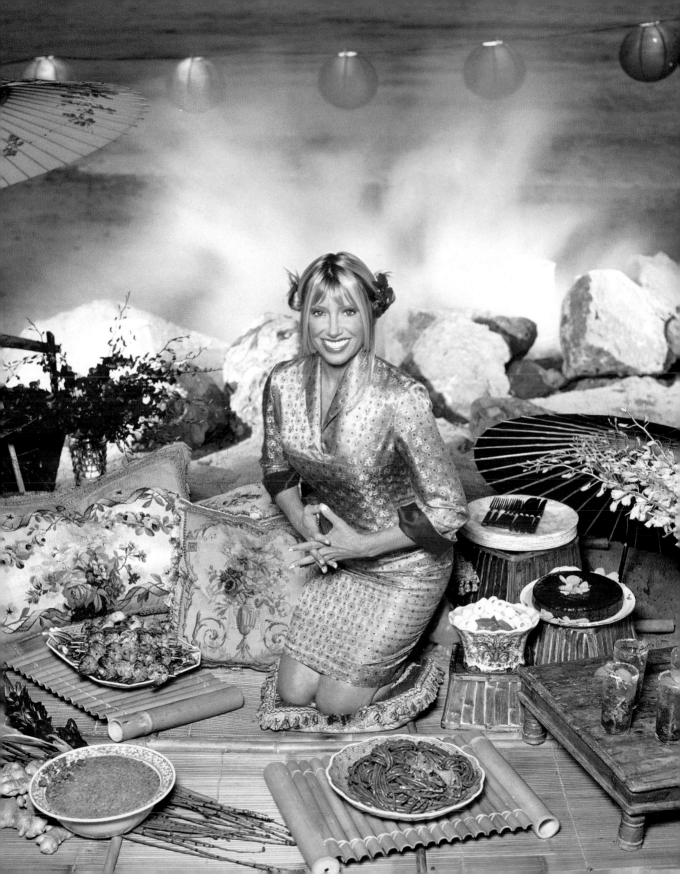

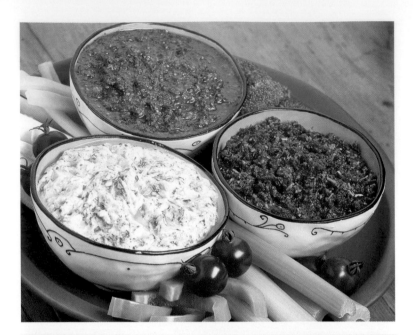

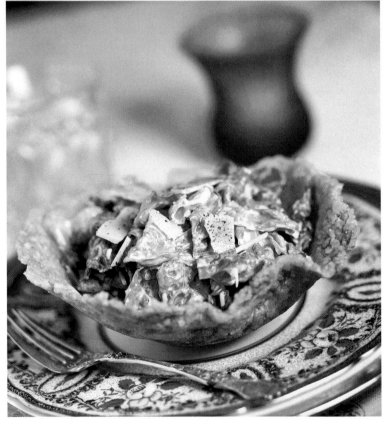

OPENING PAGE: An Oriental beach picnic, with Grilled Ginger Shrimp on Skewers, Chinese Long Beans, and Fresh Mint Tea.

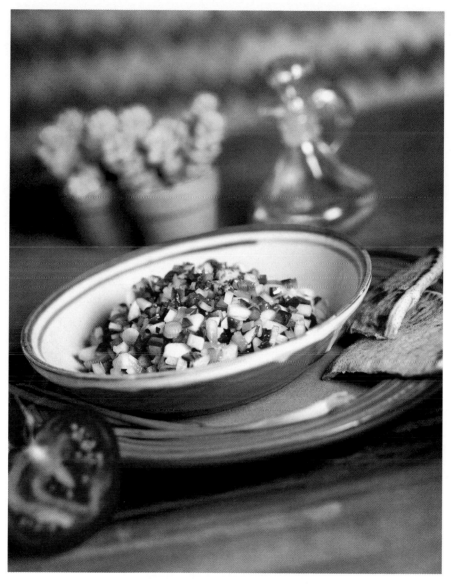

ABOVE: Israeli Salad with pita
OPPOSITE, TOP: Sun-Dried Tomato Pesto, Basil Pesto, and Artichoke Pesto
OPPOSITE, BOTTOM: Parmesan Bowls with Caesar Salad

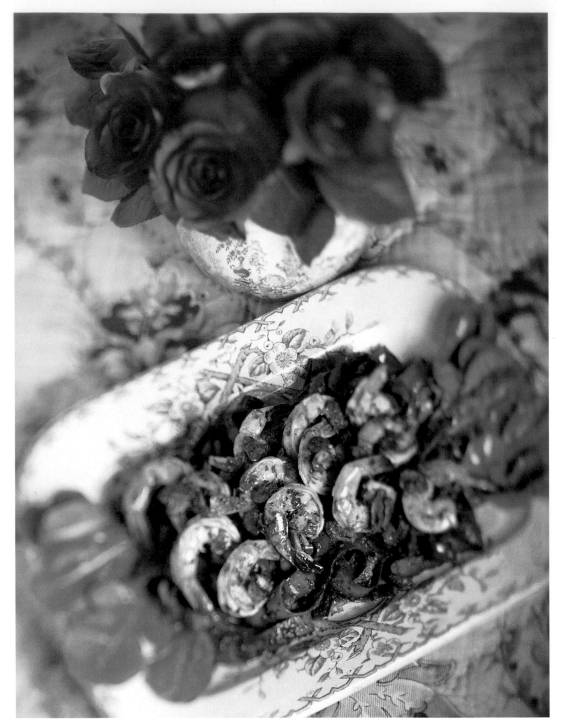

Pan-Fried Garlic Lemon Shrimp with Zucchini Pesto Noodles and Arugula

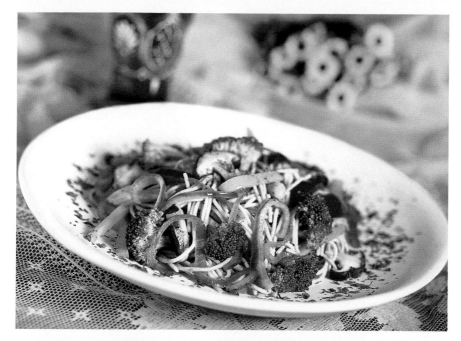

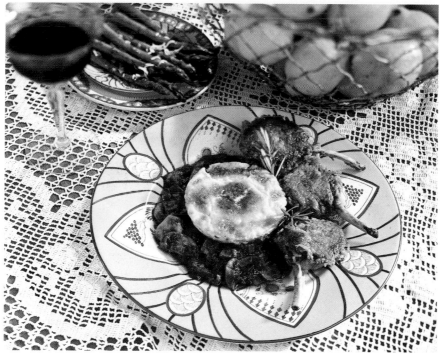

TOP: Whole-Grain Pasta Primavera

BOTTOM: Baby Lamb Chops with Parmesan Crusts, and Rosemary-Infused Savory
Custard with Tomato Mushroom Sauce

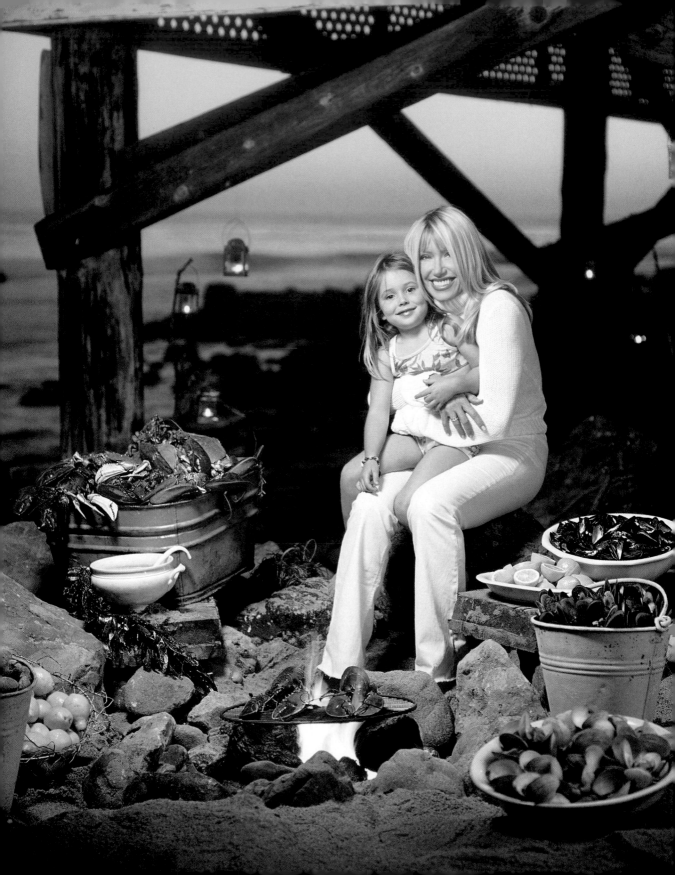

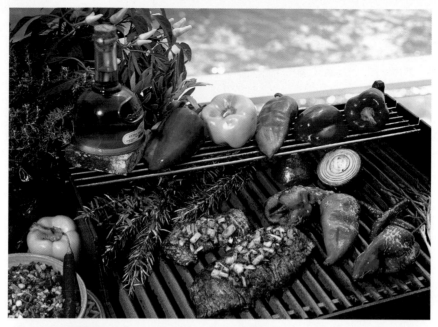

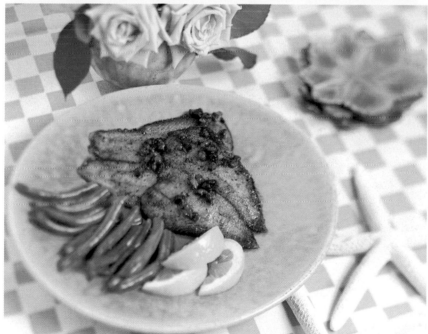

OPPOSITE : Clam Bake! Mussel Bake! Crab Bake! Lobster Bake! Can you believe that
crab, lobster, clams, and mussels dipped in melted butter is a perfectly Somersized meal?
TOP: Carne Asada de Perez with Grilled Vegetables
BOTTOM: Pan-Fried Petrale Sole with Lemon, Butter, and Caper Sauce

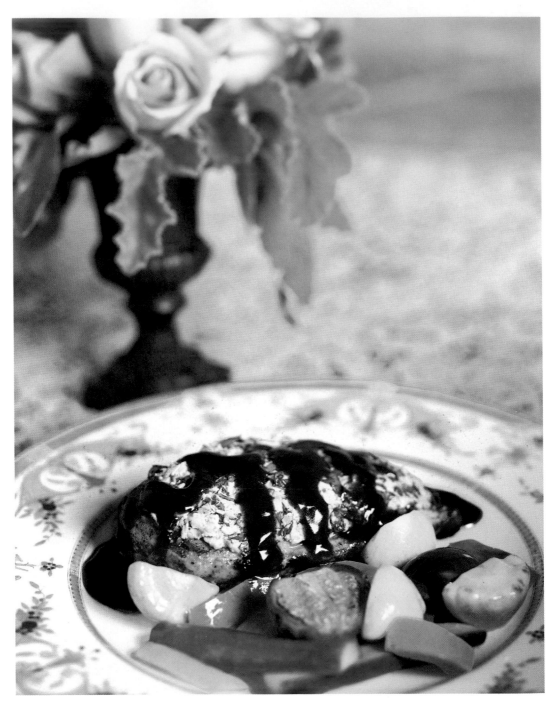

Chicken with Goat Cheese and Balsamic Syrup

or brown rice, I would make the meal predominantly a Pro/Fats meal with a small portion of pasta or rice (maybe a cup or so), rather than have a big bowl of pasta with a few pieces of meat. For me, the protein in combination with a significant amount of carbos is harder on my body than a little fat in combination with the carbos.

If I'm going to have a sandwich, I usually still have a vegetarian sandwich on whole-grain bread, but every now and then I add some avocado. The avocado has fat in it, but as long as I don't add meat as well, I generally find I do not have a problem. I also might add a little mayonnaise or olive oil, depending on the sandwich. And if I feel like a meat or tuna fish sandwich, then I usually stick to Level One and use lettuce cups instead of bread. (If I were to eat bread with meat or tuna fish, I would use only one slice and it would definitely be whole-grain bread.)

MIXING FRUIT

I still try to eat the Fruits group completely separately. The only fruit I play around with is berries, because berries are easier to digest than other fruits. They have a very high fiber content and give me very little trouble when I combine them with other foods. In Level Two I do not even think twice about eating fresh berries with whipped cream after a Pro/Fats and Veggies meal. Also, when I get tired of toast with nonfat cottage cheese or nonfat yogurt, I use a little berry jam sweetened with fruit juice, not sugar, on my toast in the morning. (Although fruit

sugar and regular sugar create a similar insulin response, most fruit-sweetened jams are not as heavily sweetened as sugared jams.) And if I just have to have pancakes, I make buckwheat or whole wheat pancakes with raspberry yogurt sauce (raspberries and nonfat yogurt) instead of maple syrup. Regular pancakes with butter and maple syrup would create a huge imbalance, whereas whole wheat, buckwheat, or multigrain pancakes served with raspberry sauce create less of an imbalance and still satisfy my craving. I also like to use berries in tarts and pies made with whole wheat crusts; certainly not Level One fare, but easier on your system than an apple tart or a pumpkin pie. And for breakfast or a snack in the afternoon I like to have fresh berries with nonfat yogurt.

I also may add a few products that are sweetened with fruit juice. At health food stores I have found a few cereals made from spelt and amaranth and kamut; flakes that are sweetened with a little fruit juice. They provide a nice change but not for every morning. Fruit juice, like sugar, creates an insulin response, but your body can handle it now, in moderation, because your cells are not overloaded with sugar.

ADDING A LITTLE SUGAR AND FUNKY FOODS

As far as sugar goes, I loosen the reins a little. I'm not quite as diligent about hunting for sugar in sauces and salad dressings. If I'm at a restaurant, I don't worry about eating a prepared blue cheese dressing on my salad, even if it has a little sugar in it. It's not enough to cause a problem for me in Level Two as long as I'm not having any Carbos. I continue to avoid gravy made with white flour and very sweet sauces, like barbecue sauce. And watch out for those thick Chinese sauces made with sugar and cornstarch. Most restaurants are happy to prepare your food without these ingredients.

If I feel like a little starch with a Pro/Fats meal, I choose parsnips over potatoes or white rice. They're not quite as starchy. I also find I can easily incorporate the foods on the Bad Combo list, such as nuts, olives, liver, avocado, and tofu.

And how about desserts? With my SomerSweet you may enjoy desserts more frequently because they are Level One, or almost Level One. Plus, they are virtually chemical free! Check out my recipes. Every now and then it's also okay to enjoy a Level Two dessert. Some desserts aren't as bad as others. I still try to stay away from the extremely sugary ones. Take a look at the sugar content in my beloved favorite, birthday cake. Just how much sugar is in a double-layer white cake with lemon filling and buttercream frosting? Two cups of sugar in the cake, a half a cup in the lemon filling, plus one more cup in the frosting. Three and a half cups of sugar! Add the copious

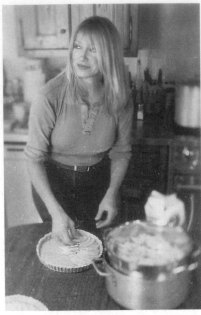

Apple Tarts with a whole wheat crust (definitely Level Two).

amounts of white flour, which are a Funky Food, the butter and eggs, Pro/Fats, and you have a poorly combined Pro/Fats, Carbos, Funky Foods concoction sure to send your system into mayhem.

Check out some of my recipes for low-sugar or no-sugar desserts. My Light Chocolate Mousse is made with cream, cocoa powder, SomerSweet, and vanilla; a much better option for Somersizing purposes. (Only the cocoa powder causes a slight imbalance because chocolate has caffeine.) But the beauty of this program is that if you really want it, you can have white cake with lemon filling and buttercream frosting—you'll just have to live back on Level One a little longer.

Another good dessert option after a Pro/Fats meal is a scoop of ice cream with fresh berries. Ice cream is often lower in sugar than other desserts and is made mostly of Pro/Fats—eggs and cream. Mine is made with SomerSweet so it's a perfect Level One dessert. If you're buying store-bought ice cream, make sure to buy the best-quality ice cream because you want it to have more cream than milk (remember, milk has carbohydrates, cream does not). Pudding, crème brûlée, and chocolate mousse are generally lower in sugar than most other desserts and do not have the addition of white flour as many pastries do. And as I mentioned, flour-less chocolate cake is a great option in Level Two, or strawberries dipped in chocolate with freshly whipped cream!

You really can eat these desserts and maintain your weight if you are Somersizing properly. Check out my recipes for desserts. You'll be knocked out by how great they are. They are all made with SomerSweet and I use whole wheat pastry flour instead of white flour. I used to apologize for my desserts made with artificial sweetener because although technically these desserts are Level One fare, I didn't want you eating chemical-laden desserts after every meal, thinking they were perfectly okay since they have no sugar. Now that we have Somer-Sweet, I have included lots of desserts so that you have an alternative to a sugary dessert while you are diligently sticking to your Level One guidelines.

YOU'RE IN CONTROL

As far as Level Two goes, you are in control. Maybe you don't miss the sweets as much as you miss the bread. Then save your treats for a great baguette or a chewy sourdough roll. Or if it's white pasta you're craving, eat mostly Level One meals and then indulge yourself with a little pasta fix. It's up to you. For me, the whole-grain pasta is so good that I don't ever feel deprived eating it instead of white pasta. Sometimes I even bring it to my favorite Italian restaurants and ask the kitchen to use it, instead of white pasta. They never seem to mind, as long as I pay full price for my dish. I still stay away from meat sauce with my whole-grain pasta because the combination makes me bloat.

How you choose your imbalances depends on many factors. How many imbalances have you had today and how big were your imbalances today? How many big imbalances have you had this week? Don't get cocky with your new figure! The pounds can creep their way back on to your body if you're not careful.

Beware of the slipups. It usually starts with one dessert, which leads to another, and then another. Before you know it you've started adding bad combinations and a little white flour here and there. Your body will signal you with warning signs. Learn to listen to them! If you start craving sugar and carbohydrates, it means you are eating too much of them. That's what happens; the more sugar you eat, the more you crave. Then come the energy dips, the extra pounds, and don't forget about the damage you're doing on the inside to your healthy cells. And remember, the best way to take away a sugar craving is to eat a Pro/Fat because Pro/Fats help to stabilize blood sugar. So next time you have a craving for sugar or carbohydrates, eat a piece of cheese and it should help the problem. All in all, if you notice signs that your body is starting to crave sugar again, go back to Level One until you get rid of the problem. Stay on top of the new you. Take care of your body.

I also want to mention a few words about portion control. On Level One you may eat as much as you want as long as you are fol-lowing *all* the Level One guidelines. (That means technically you can gorge yourself and not gain weight, although I'm sure you did not end up overeating, because your appetite was fully satisfied with wholesome, nutritious foods.) In Level Two, you must consider limiting your portions when you are creating imbalances. You can't have it both ways—the bonus of Level One is that you can eat as much as you want. The bonus of Level Two is that you have more variety, but you must limit your portions moderately.

WINE AND CHOCOLATE

Recent studies have shown that red wine has been proven to have beneficial effects on the heart by helping to keep your arteries clear. I have incorporated it, in moderation, in Level Two. Remember, your body accepts wine as sugar, so don't overdo it. Some people find they can enjoy a glass or two of wine with their meals without having any problems. However, wine combined with other imbalances can add up to too much sugar. Keep those insulin levels intact or you'll end up back where you started. I drink wine a couple times a week and I use it freely in many of my recipes. It creates only a slight imbalance because most of the alcohol is cooked off in the process. In fact, I cook with wine even in Level One, because it wonderfully enhances the flavor of my meals and does not seem to disrupt my system. If you are doing well on Level One, you should not have a problem doing the same.

Now for chocolate . . . my great love! I can't seem to live without chocolate; and I don't have to. Dark chocolate (more than 60 percent cocoa) is relatively low in sugar and does not create a huge imbalance. And now I have my SomerSweet Chocolate Truffles, which create only a tiny imbalance! (Available at SuzanneSomers.com.) The best time to eat chocolate is on an empty stomach, perhaps a couple of squares in the afternoon. And I have many sinful low-sugar desserts made from dark chocolate that are perfect for Level Two.

You will continue to use all of the recipes in Level One for Level Two. I have included a few recipes specific to Level Two for your enjoyment. In addition, check out all the great recipes in *Eat Great, Lose Weight* and *Get Skinny on Fabulous Food*. Good luck in this new phase. You have such freedom in Level Two, I just know you will love it. Any questions you have will be answered by your own body as you experiment with Level Two. Eating this way is truly a pleasure and I'm sure you will be the envy of all of your friends who can't believe what wonderful foods you eat and still manage to keep your beautiful figure.

MEAL PLANS, LEVEL TWO

From week to week my meal plans will vary greatly on Level Two. I am sharing this particular week of meals with you because it was a good model week for me in terms of balancing my Pro/Fats and Carbos and getting plenty of Fruits and Veggies. You will see that there is a combination of Level One meals and Level Two meals. Remember, your body may be able to handle more or less imbalance depending on your unique metabolism. I can handle about this many imbalances and still maintain my weight. To help you see how I choose my treats, I have put an asterisk next to the items that are Level Two, with a brief explanation regarding the imbalance.

SUNDAY

9:00 BREAKFAST
Grilled Onion Frittata (p. 137)
Decaf coffee

1:00 LUNCH
Sliced gyros served over lettuce with
    tomato and garlic cucumber sauce
1 piece of whole wheat pita bread★
*(★I combined whole wheat pita with a Pro/Fats
    and Veggies meal)*

3:00 SNACK
A hard-boiled egg

7:00 DINNER
Grilled chicken breast
Steamed broccoli and cauliflower tossed
    in garlic vinaigrette
Green salad with garlic vinaigrette
A glass of red wine★
One square of dark chocolate★
(★wine and chocolate)

MONDAY

BREAKFAST
(9:00) Mango
(9:30) Rye toast with berry jam★
Decaf coffee
*(★Berry jam creates a slight imbalance with my
    toast)*

1:30 LUNCH
Warm goat cheese salad with chicken,
    pine nuts, and sun-dried tomatoes★

Flourless chocolate cake★
*(★I added pine nuts to my salad. Plus the Level
    Two dessert has a little sugar and chocolate.)*

7:30 DINNER
Lemony Chicken Burgers (p. 221)
Steamed green beans
Butter lettuce salad with balsamic
    vinaigrette

TUESDAY

7:30 BREAKFAST
Cantaloupe
Decaf coffee

12:00 LUNCH
Stir-fried vegetables with brown rice★
(★I used oil in a Carbos and Veggies meal.)

3:00 SNACK
A piece of cheddar cheese

7:00 DINNER
Roasted yellow pepper soup
Green salad with zucchini and shaved
    Parmesan
Braised lamb shank

WEDNESDAY

7:30 BREAKFAST
Eggs Baked in Tomatoes and Red
    Peppers (p. 136)
One slice whole-grain toast with
    butter★
Decaf coffee
*(★I combined whole-grain toast with a Pro/Fats
    meal)*

1:00 LUNCH
Chicken Breasts with Sage
    (p. 223)
Cabbage salad
Steamed green beans

4:00 SNACK
Dawn's Deviled Eggs (p. 129)

7:30 DINNER
Jalapeño Chili (p. 240) topped with
cheddar cheese, sour cream, and
cilantro★
Green salad with red wine vinaigrette
Whipped cream with fresh berries★

(*I added a few garbanzo beans and navy beans to
the chili. Dessert was barely an imbalance at all
because I did not sweeten the whipped cream
and the berries are fine for Level Two.)*

THURSDAY

7:30 BREAKFAST
Whole wheat toast with tomatoes and
basil★

(*I put a little olive oil on my toast in this Carbos
and Veggies meal.)*

10:00 SNACK
An orange

12:30 LUNCH
Whole-Grain Pasta Primavera (p. 187)
with Parmesan cheese
Green salad with romaine, red cabbage,
celery, and red wine vinaigrette
A glass of red wine★

(*I combined oil, walnuts, and Parmesan cheese
with my Carbos and Veggies, plus a glass of
wine.)*

6:30 DINNER
Baby Back Pork Ribs (p. 230)
Sautéed Spinach with Garlic, Lemon,
and Olive Oil (p. 201)
Steamed asparagus

FRIDAY

7:00 BREAKFAST
Buckwheat pancakes★

Decaf coffee

(*These pancakes create a moderate imbalance.)*

1:00 LUNCH
Rotisserie chicken
Caesar Salad (no croutons)

6:30 DINNER
Beef Stir-Fry (p. 243)
Brown rice★

(*I had a small serving of brown rice with a
Pro/Fats and Veggies meal.)*

SATURDAY

BREAKFAST
(8:00) Fruit smoothie
(8:30) Whole-grain toast with berry
jam★

(*Berry jam creates a slight imbalance with my
Carbos.)*

1:00 LUNCH
Roasted peppers with pecorino
cheese★
Grilled whole-grain bread★
Baked garlic★
Cannelini bean dip★
Green beans with garlic★
Tricolore salad with balsamic vinai-
grette★

(*I combined oil and cheese with Carbos & Veggies.)*

7:00 DINNER
Rosemary Roast Loin of Pork (p. 229)
Caramelized Fennel (p. 196)
Wild rice
Israeli Salad (p. 175)
A glass of red wine★
Molten Chocolate Cakes (p. 259)
whipped cream★

(*The wild rice, chocolate cakes, and wine create a
slight imbalance with this dinner.)*

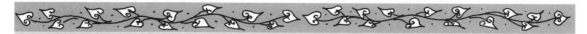

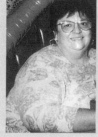

before

Dear Suzanne,

If you were near me, I would give you such a hug. I am a success story. A big success!

I ordered the "Somersize" package from the Shopping Channel here in Canada February 2000. My doctor had been begging me to lose weight because of high blood pressure. I weighed in at 277. I am only 5 feet 4 inches. I am 58 years old and have been fat most of my life.

My sister and I started to follow your program. The pounds simply melted off me. They melted so fast that my doctor was concerned. He asked to see the book. He was impressed with it and told me: "Anyone who says No to Funky Foods is OK in my book!"

I feel terrific. I have energy to spare. The best news is that so far I have lost 66 pounds. There are more pounds to come off. I do not feel hungry, except when I miss a meal (which is very seldom). I am a great example of how well this program works. So many people ask me how I do it. I tell them I do not diet, I follow the program and it works. Thank you again, Suzanne.

Cecile Bertrand

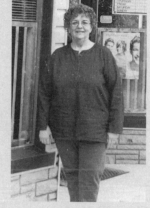

after

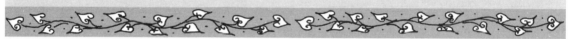

As my son, Bruce, says, "Level Two is just eating." And he's right. You don't ever have to deny yourself anything. I just can't indulge myself every time I have a craving, but I do it often enough so that I never feel deprived.

With your new figure and your improved health comes a renewed sense of self-confidence. You set out to achieve a goal and you have attained it. You should be proud of yourself. Enjoy your meals, enjoy your new body, and enjoy knowing that you are giving your body the nutritious foods it needs to thrive and ward off disease. Somer-

sizing has truly been a liberating experience for me. I am finally in control of my weight rather than my weight being in control of me. I hope in sharing it with you that your life has been enhanced in some way, either through losing a few pounds or learning some new tricks in the kitchen.

SEND ME YOUR STORIES

My favorite part about putting together this book was reading all the success stories from people just like you. I can't tell you how gratifying it is for me to hear about the weight you've lost and about how you've learned to cook some fabulous new recipes. Please write to me and let me know how you are doing on the program. I would love to hear from you. And if you like, pass along any good recipes of your own!

Suzanne Somers
c/o Crown Publishers
299 Park Avenue
New York, NY 10171

Additionally, take a look at my Web site at www.suzannesomers.com or Somersize.com. It will be updated constantly to answer all of your questions. Check it out!

THIRTEEN

Frequently Asked Somersize Questions

After writing three books and making count-less appearances where I talk about Somersiz-ing, you can imagine that I have heard a lot of questions from people who are really inspired by Somersizing but have some ques-tions about the program. In *Eat, Cheat, and Melt the Fat Away* I want to take the opportu-nity to answer some of the most frequently asked questions I've heard throughout the years from curious Somersizers. Now that you have finished this book and are ready to make some of my delicious, perfectly Somer-sized recipes, I hope that this section will answer some of your own questions!

Can I use ketchup on Level One?

Ketchup is usually sweetened with some form of sugar. It is important in the early stages of Somersizing to eliminate all sugars so you get rid of all cravings.

Can I have sugar-free Jell-O and/or sugar-free puddings?

Sugar-free Jell-O is okay, but you should be aware that it contains aspartame and is loaded with chemicals. When you need a dessert fix, it is great with whipped cream, but I would eat it sparingly. Sugar-free Jell-O can be eaten after a Pro/Fats meal or a Carbos meal. Sugar-free pudding has corn-starch and lots of carbs. Try my sugarless desserts made with SomerSweet.

Can I have mayonnaise, oil, and salad dress-ings?

You can't have oil and mayo with Carbos, but you can have them with protein, which is chicken, meat, or fish. For instance, a chicken salad with mayo would be perfect.

Where does buttermilk fit into Somersizing?

Buttermilk is a Funky Food because it has fat and carbohydrates, just like whole milk or low-fat milk. In this book I have added it to the Funky Foods list.

Can I have fat-free cheese with my Carbos?

Technically, yes, but check the ingredients list because many of these products are filled with chemicals your body does not want or need.

Can I have tofu?

Tofu has protein, fat, and carbs, so it is a Funky Food . . . technically. However, there are many people who use it in Pro/Fats meals with oil, cheese, and veggies or in Carbos with Veggies meals and they have no problem. It is a very minor imbalance. If you are doing well on Level One, you should not have a problem adding tofu. It is fine for Level Two.

I am craving sweets. What do you suggest?

Eat a piece of cheese to stop the craving. Also, check my Web site because I am developing supplements to help stop sugar cravings.

I have been unable to locate any whole wheat pasta, cereal, or bread that does not have some fat. Even Grape Nuts has ¹/₅ gram of fat.

Don't worry about the fat content listed per serving in the nutritional panel. Look at the ingredients list and make sure there is no *added* fat. Many grains have minimal amounts of fat that will not create a problem. Grape Nuts are perfect for Somersizing. As for bread, Ezekial brand has no fat or sugar. If you can't find it, try whole wheat pita.

I have found that almost all the whole wheat breads have molasses or honey in them. Is there a certain brand you recommend? Will the amounts of molasses and honey in these breads throw me off track?

Unfortunately, most whole wheat breads in standard grocery stores have sugar of some form or another. If you have a bakery in your city, ask them for a multigrain bread that has no sugar, molasses, honey, or any other form of sugar. It might cost a little more, but the flavor is so much better and more delicious, I'm sure you'll find that it's worth it. If you still can't find any free of sweeteners, limit your intake to reduce the effect.

Are dried fruits allowed?

Yes, but only sparingly because the sugar content has been concentrated during the drying process. Limit your intake in Level One.

Can I have juice?

By the time you make juice from fruit you have taken out almost all the nutrition and are left with fruit sugar. Technically, if you are drinking juice alone, you may have it in the same way you eat fruit alone. However, many juices are very high in natural fruit sugar and I recommend you drink them sparingly. The whole fruit also contains fiber, which helps to reduce the effects of insulin. Sometimes on Level One it's great to enjoy a Popsicle made from fruit and fruit juice only. Just beware of eating too many products with concentrated fruit juice because it will make your insulin spike.

Can I have a veggie burger?

Vegetarian burgers are often made of soy, vegetables, and grains. Soy and nuts are both Funky Foods because they contain fat and carbohydrates. However, if you are doing well on Level One and really want a veggie burger, it probably will not create that much of an imbalance. On Level Two they are fine.

Can I use artificial flavorings and extracts in foods?

Yes, but when you start eating real foods, you learn to enjoy nature's real flavors.

Can I use artificial sweeteners?

I have done research on artificial sweeteners such as aspartame and I feel very strongly that this is a dangerous chemical and should be eliminated for health reasons, not for weight loss purposes. Many Somersizers eat and drink products with artificial sweeteners (aspartame and saccharin) because they need something sweet during Level One. Now I have SomerSweet, an all-natural sugar substitute that won't spike your insulin and is

not received by the body as a carbohydrate. It's a miracle!

What about low-fat dairy products?

Low-fat milk is not included in this program because it contains fat and carbohydrates. Low-fat cheese contains less fat and also some carbohydrates. Full-fat cheese tastes so much better and is perfectly okay on Level One. Nonfat dairy products have no fat and only carbohydrates, so you can have them as a Carbo on Level One.

What can I have for a snack?

You can have little pieces of meat, cheese, fruit, hard-boiled eggs, veggies with blue cheese dip.

Can I have salad dressing?

Yes! The great thing about Somersizing is that you can have the oil and the fats. Watch out for commercially prepared dressings that have sugar or some type of starch or thickener in them. You can have salad dressings with oil and fat when you are eating a Pro/Fats and Veggies meal. If you are having a Carbos and Veggies meal, your dressing can have no fat.

Do I have to drink a lot of water?

I highly recommend you drink 8–10 glasses of water a day. But try not to drink with your meals because water can dilute your digestive juices, which slows down the digestive process. Your stomach acids are strongest right before you begin a new meal. When you eat, the acids break down the food quickly and pass it from the stomach. If you drink a big glass of water before your meal, these gastric juices become diluted and are less effective at breaking down the food. Therefore, if you must drink with your meal, eat a portion of your food before you drink anything so as not to dilute the strength of the gastric juices. It's best to drink your 8–10 glasses between meals.

What kinds of foods should I order in a restaurant?

Pro/Fats and Veggies are the easiest to order in restaurants because there is so much variety. I find that Carbos meals are more restrictive.

What about whole wheat?

Many people see wheat flour on an ingredients list and assume it is whole wheat flour. This is incorrect. White flour can originate as wheat flour; it's just been stripped of its nutrients and its color. You must look for whole wheat flour, whole wheat, cracked whole wheat, or stone ground whole wheat.

You may also have other whole-grain pastas and breads (remember, no fat or sugar added). They include amaranth, barley, bran, brown rice, buckwheat, durum wheat, farina, kamut, millet, oats, pumpernickel, rye, spelt, or lavash bread (or any combination of the above). Semolina is not included in this group because it is "the purified middlings of hard wheat (as durum) used for pasta (as macaroni or spaghetti)." When something has been "purified," it is usually bleached, as in "bleached wheat flour"—white flour. So, when the label says "durum wheat semolina" or "durum semolina," they mean the bleached inner part of what used to be whole wheat. Look for durum *whole* wheat.

What cereals can I have?

Regular Grape Nuts, Puffed Wheat, and Shredded Wheat are fine. Grape Nuts Flakes have added sugar so you need to avoid them. Don't get confused by reading the grams of sugar on the nutritional panel. For instance, Grape Nuts and Grape Nuts Flakes show the same sugar content in the nutritional panel, but regular Grape Nuts' sugar comes from malted barley and Grape Nuts Flakes have added sugar . . . so no Flakes. Rule of thumb, read the ingredients list for added sugars and fats. Cheerios have added sugar and modified cornstarch, but I enjoy them in Level Two without a problem.

How much should I be eating? Do I have to count calories or fat?

Do not count fat grams, carbs, or calories or weigh anything. Follow the Level One guidelines and eat what you want until comfortably full. Try to eat a wide variety of foods each day.

Can I eat any meat I want?

Yes, just make sure it is not cured with sugar. (Pork is most often the culprit.) Watch out for cold cuts and be sure to read the ingredients list.

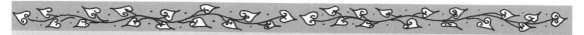

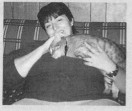

before

Dear Suzanne,

I wanted to thank you for your wonderful way to eat. I have lost 139 pounds and am still losing. I weighed 295 pounds, and now I weigh 156 pounds. I have a rare muscle disorder called Dystonia. It is in the Parkinson family—there is no cure and it is progressive. I had gained 93 pounds and was unable to lose at all. My weight just kept going up. The doctors wouldn't even talk to me about a diet because it would lead to muscle loss. On your diet, or your way of eating, I like to call it, I lost all of my weight and didn't lose my muscle because of the way I was eating. I have lost this weight with no exercise. Most of the time I have been flat on my back.

My doctors have really been just overwhelmed by this. They are telling their other patients about your book. I am able to help transfer myself now to my wheelchair and even roll myself where before I could not. I have also been able to even come off my blood pressure medicine. You have really helped me in a time of need. Thank you so very much.

Sincerely,
Angie Burcham

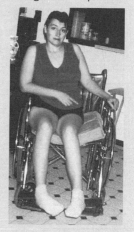

after

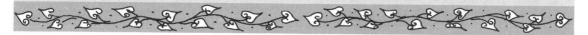

Should I use margarine?

Even though margarine is listed as a Pro/Fat, I avoid it because of the trans fatty acids. Also try to avoid any food that has the word *hydrogenated* on the package. Adding hydrogen to fat makes it a cheap filler for the producer. Unfortunately, it raises your LDL cholesterol (bad) and lowers your HDL cholesterol (the good one that helps get rid of the bad).

What about egg whites?

Even though they are fat free, do not eat them on Level One with a Carbos meal.

They are still considered a protein. Since proteins and carbs digest at different rates, you will be combining improperly.

Why can I use olive oil and I can't have olives?

You can have olive oil because it is a pure fat, but olives contain fat and carbohydrates. Olives are fine on Level Two.

Can I have yogurt?

Nonfat yogurt is a Carbo and perfectly fine on Level One. Choose nonfat plain yogurt and sweeten it with SomerSweet and vanilla extract. Sprinkle a few Grape Nuts on top.

Is yogurt a carb or a fat? And can I have the yogurt with fruit in it?

Nonfat yogurt is a carbohydrate. Low-fat or whole-milk yogurt has carbs and fat, which makes them Funky Foods. Yogurt with fruit at the bottom is usually loaded with sugar. Nonfat plain yogurt with fresh berries is a very minor imbalance.

Are peas considered a Carbo or a Veggie?

Peas are listed in the Carbo group.

What about beans?

All beans (except green beans) are grouped with the Carbos for the purpose of Somer-sizing.

Can I have no-sugar-added, full-fat ice cream?

Yes. But watch out for chemicals . . . you won't gain weight from them, but they are not good for you. Try my Vanilla Bean Ice Cream (p. 250). It's made with cream (not milk) and SomerSweet (not artificial sweetener).

If I want coffee, am I limited to decaf coffee?

Caffeinated drinks are stimulants and cause a surge of insulin all on their own. When you combine your foods correctly, you'll get a natural energy boost instead of an artificial caffeine buzz.

Can I use cream in my coffee?

If you've had a Pro/Fats meal, use cream (check the label and make sure it's just cream, not nonfat dry milk). If you've had a Carbos meal, use skim milk.

Is Coffee-mate creamer allowed?

The first two ingredients in Coffee-mate creamer are corn syrup and vegetable oil, so you should not use it. Use cream in your coffee for a Pro/Fats meal or nonfat milk for a Carbos meal. You may also add SomerSweet.

Is half-and-half allowed?

Half-and-half is a combination of milk and cream. Because of the milk, half-and-half has trace amounts of carbohydrates. You would be better off using cream.

Is it better for me to eat my Carbos in the morning, or doesn't it matter?

The earlier in the day the better because you are more likely to burn them off as fuel. Remember, carbohydrates equal sugar equals energy. You don't want your last meal of the day to be fuel, because most likely you are going to go to bed shortly after. If fuel is not burned off, it has the potential to be stored as fat even if it is a whole grain or fruit.

How much fruit can I eat? Is there a limit?

I don't give you any limits on how much fruit you should eat; but remember, fruit is a natural sugar. If you are eating a lot of fruit and find you are not losing weight, I would try cutting back to see if that helps. I usually eat fruit in the morning and occasionally as a snack in the afternoon. And don't forget to eat fruit on an empty stomach.

Are there fruits I should avoid?

Even though bananas are high in potassium, they are also very high in starch. That is why they are a Funky Food. With all the other fruits you can eat, you won't miss them. Berries are very high in fiber and therefore cause only a slight imbalance when eaten with other foods. If you are doing well on Level One, you may enjoy berries with whipped cream after a Pro/Fats meal. On Level Two, I sometimes use all-fruit-juice-sweetened berry jam on my whole-grain toast in the morning.

I'm not a breakfast eater. Is it important to have breakfast?

If you skip breakfast, your body has gone sometimes over twelve hours without any food. By the time you eat lunch your body may hang on to every morsel for fear it might not get food again. The best way to increase your metabolism is to eat. Try to have a little something for breakfast.

Is it okay to have the sugar-free lemonade drinks like Country Time and Crystal Light?

Yes, but do know that most sugar-free drinks contain aspartame, which has been known to cause brain damage in laboratory rats. Personally, I try to stay away from all chemicals and drink as much water as possible. But if you are craving a soft drink, the caffeine-free, sugar-free ones are the best.

Can I have the sugar-free hard candies?

Yes, but only in moderation. They are filled with chemicals, so you are trading sugar for chemicals.

How about sugar-free chocolate candy?

I understand we all have sugar cravings, and these are certainly better than eating candy with sugar. Use them in moderation because of the chemicals in sugar-free products. A better alternative is my Chocolate Truffles recipe (p. 263). Yum!

Is peanut butter allowed?

It is made from peanuts, which are Funky Foods. When you get to Level Two, you can enjoy it in moderation.

Are nuts okay to eat?

Nuts are a Funky Food. When you get to Level Two, you can enjoy them in moderation.

Can I have pickles?

Sure, as long as they are dill pickles and not sweet pickles. As with all foods, check the ingredients to make sure there is no added sugar.

Can I eat cheese anytime I feel I need a snack, or do I have to wait a certain amount of time after a Carbos meal?

Cheese is an excellent snack, but you must wait three hours after a Carbos meal. Otherwise, the fat from the cheese, along with the carbs still in your system, could cause your body to accept both substances as a carbohydrate.

Are pumpernickel bagels okay to eat? If so, what can I have on them?

Read the ingredients on the bagel packaging to make sure they have not added any sugar or white flour. If they are made from pumpernickel flour, they are fine for a Carbos meal; but on Level One do not use cream cheese or butter. Try nonfat cottage cheese, nonfat ricotta cheese, sliced tomatoes, onions, and fresh basil. Many people use nonfat cream cheese, but I have found these products to be filled with starches and chemicals and I don't recommend them.

Can I have Chinese food? I know I can't have the rice, but what can I have?

Eating in a Chinese restaurant is very difficult because they use sugary sauces as a base in most of their preparations. Some Chinese restaurants are offering brown rice and steamed vegetables, or you could order stir-fried vegetables with chicken, meat, or fish and ask them to cook it in oil and soy sauce only. Personally, I would also ask them to eliminate MSG because it's a chemical.

What about soy milk and other soy products, like soy nuts?

Nonfat soy milk is included in the Carbos group because it has carbs without fat. Regular soy milk, tofu, and soy nuts are considered Funky Foods because they contain protein, fat, and carbs. If you are a strict vegetarian and you need additional protein sources, I make an exception with tofu and soy products because the carbohydrate content is not terribly high. In addition, in Level Two, these are some of the first foods I encourage you to put back into your eating plan because soy has such important nutrients.

Can juice be used in smoothies for Level One?

Yes, just make sure it does not have any added sugar.

About half an hour after I have a Pro/Fats meal I am hungry again. Am I doing something wrong?

Eat more! Have larger portions. Eat until you feel satisfied. Keep hard-boiled eggs in the fridge to help fill you up after a meal.

Can I have chocolate?

On Level Two you may enjoy dark chocolate in moderation. It must be at least 60 percent cocoa. I like Valhrona, but there are many others. I'm developing one with Somer-Sweet, so check my Web site in the future. SuzanneSomers.com or Somersize.com.

Can I use brown rice pasta?

Yes, because it is made from the whole grain.

Is gum allowed? If so, what kind?

Sugar-free gum is allowed, but don't overdo it. Sorbitol, NutraSweet, and saccharin are chemicals, and the most healthy choice is to eliminate them.

Why is liver not allowed on this program?

Liver has protein, fat, and carbohydrate, making it a Funky Food. You may enjoy it on Level Two without a problem.

What is celery root? Where do I find it in the grocery store and in what form?

Celery root is a large brown root usually with a few celery stalks coming out the top. Look near the other roots, like horseradish and parsnips. When in doubt, ask your produce manager where it is. If they don't carry it, ask them to special-order it for you.

I am on the drug Tamoxifen. Can that be slowing down my weight loss?

Absolutely. Tamoxifen interferes with your hormones; and when there is hormonal imbalance, there can be weight gain.

I just found out I'm diabetic. Is Somersizing good for me?

Diabetes is a serious condition and you should check with your doctor. I've received hundreds of letters from diabetics who say this plan is a miracle for them, which makes sense because Somersizing eliminates sugar and sugar elevates your insulin levels.

Part Two

THE

SOMERSIZE

RECIPES

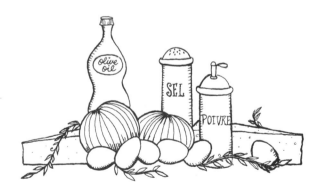

Breakfast and Brunch

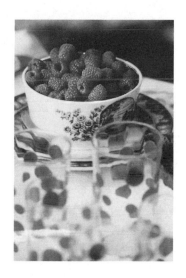

Somersize Zucchini Muffins

MAKES 24

These awesome muffins were inspired by a fellow Somersizer, Jennifer Blackwell. They make a perfect Level One Carbos breakfast and keep you full all morning long. Thanks for sending your recipe, Jennifer!

2½ cups nonfat milk
4 tablespoons SomerSweet or saccharin
2 tablespoons vanilla extract
1 tablespoon orange extract
¼ teaspoon cinnamon
¼ teaspoon nutmeg
2 cups quick-cooking oats
2 cups All-Bran cereal (see Note)
2 medium zucchini, shredded (about 2 cups)

32 ounces nonfat plain yogurt
4 cups whole wheat flour
2½ teaspoons baking soda
2½ teaspoons baking powder
1 teaspoon grated lemon zest
2 tablespoons plus 2 teaspoons lemon juice
3 tablespoons grated orange zest

Preheat oven to 400 degrees.

Heat milk in a saucepan until just boiling. Add Somersweet (or saccharin), vanilla, orange extract, cinnamon, and nutmeg. Remove from heat and set aside.

In a large mixing bowl combine oats, All-Bran, zucchini, and yogurt. Add hot milk and mix to form a batter. Stir in flour, and add baking powder, baking soda, lemon zest, lemon juice, and orange zest. Stir well.

Scoop batter into nonstick muffin pans.

Bake at 400 degrees for 8 minutes, then reduce heat to 350 and bake for an additional 20–25 minutes, or until golden brown.

When the muffins have cooled, wrap those that will not be eaten within a day or two individually in plastic wrap, place in a storage bag, and freeze.

Note
All-Bran has trace amounts of sugar and will not create an imbalance.

Dawn's Deviled Eggs

PRO/FATS AND VEGGIES—LEVEL ONE

MAKES 10

My good friend Barry Manilow has a wonderful cook named Dawn. These are her delicious deviled eggs. Her original recipe includes avocado, which makes the filling green. Try it that way for Level Two.

5 hard-boiled eggs, halved lengthwise
1 tablespoon minced scallion, white and
   light green parts
1 large jalapeño pepper, seeded and minced

Juice from 1 lime
1 tablespoon mayonnaise
$\frac{1}{2}$ teaspoon kosher salt, or to taste
red chili flakes for garnish

Remove the yolks from the whites. Set the whites aside. Mash the yolks in a bowl with a fork. Add the scallion, jalapeño, lime juice, mayonnaise, and salt. Add more mayonnaise to reach desired consistency. Mash with a fork until blended. Using a teaspoon, carefully stuff whites with yolk mixture, mounding the tops.

For extra heat, garnish with red chili flakes.

For Level Two
Add 1 whole mashed avocado to the egg yolk mixture.

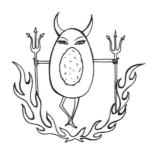

Mozzarella Marinara

PRO/FATS AND VEGGIES—LEVEL ONE

SERVES 4–6

Traditionally, mozzarella marinara is made by coating mozzarella with egg and bread crumbs. I Somersized it by coating it in Parmesan cheese instead. It's bubbly and melty and covered in a delicious tomato sauce. Indulge, guilt free!

1 pound mozzarella cheese
2 eggs, lightly beaten
¾ cup freshly grated Parmesan cheese

1 recipe Sweet Tomato Sauce (p. 235) or
    your favorite marinara

Preheat the broiler.

Slice the cheese across the width into slices ½ inch thick. Dip each slice of cheese in the beaten egg, then coat in Parmesan cheese. Place the prepared cheese slices on a plate and freeze them until just before you are ready to cook them.

Warm the tomato sauce in a small saucepan.

Arrange the frozen cheese slices on a baking sheet. Place the baking sheet under the broiler for 2–3 minutes, until the cheese starts to bubble and turn golden brown. Carefully flip over each cheese slice with a spatula and brown the other side.

Place each slice on a plate and top with warm tomato sauce. Serve immediately.

Egg Crêpes

PRO/FATS AND VEGGIES—LEVEL ONE

SERVES 4

Alan's mother used to make these delicious egg crêpes. She'd roll and then slice them to make the most divine Egg Crêpe Noodles in Chicken Broth (p. 162). You can also stuff the crêpes with a variety of fillings (pp. 132–134). Now Alan is the master egg crêpe maker. The grandchildren love them. I'm sure this recipe will stay in the family for many generations to come.

6 eggs
Salt and freshly ground black pepper

Butter

In a mixing bowl, lightly beat the eggs. Season with salt and pepper. Heat a crêpe or omelette pan over medium to medium high heat and lightly coat the bottom and sides with butter.

Using a ladle, put enough egg in the pan to make a thin coating. When it sets, lift up with a spatula, being careful not to tear the crêpe, and turn. Cook one more minute and then slide the crêpe out of the pan and onto a dish. Continue making egg crêpes in this way until you have used all the batter. Stack the crêpes as you would pancakes. Choose one of the crêpe fillings on pp. 132–134, or make one up of your own.

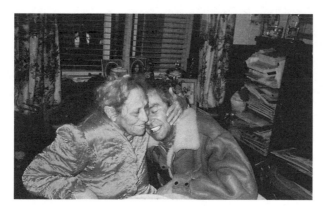

Show me a man who loves his mother, and I'll show you a man who is a great husband. Alan with his mother.

Egg Crêpes with Wild Mushroom Filling

PRO/FATS AND VEGGIES—LEVEL ONE

MAKES 6–8 CRÊPES

Alan's mother's famous egg crêpes stuffed with my wild mushroom filling make a divine lunch! Also try the Spinach and Ricotta and Ground Beef fillings for a trio of flavors, topped with Creamy Parmesan Sauce (p. 135).

1 tablespoon butter
1 pound assorted mushrooms, thinly sliced
    (shiitake, oyster, crimini, or button)
Salt and freshly ground black pepper

1 recipe Egg Crêpes (p. 131)
1 recipe Creamy Parmesan Sauce (p. 135)
    (optional)

Heat a medium sauté pan on medium. Melt the butter and add mushrooms. Cook the mushrooms until soft and tender, about 15–20 minutes. Season with salt and pepper.

Lay each egg crêpe flat, then place about ⅓ cup filling across the width. Roll the crêpe burrito style, and serve with the folded side down. Top with Creamy Parmesan Sauce, if desired.

Egg Crêpes with Spinach and Ricotta Filling

PRO/FATS AND VEGGIES—LEVEL ONE

MAKES 6–8 CRÊPES

2 tablespoons olive oil
3 cloves garlic, minced
8 ounces frozen chopped spinach, thawed
    and drained
1 pound ricotta cheese

Salt and freshly ground black pepper
1/8 teaspoon nutmeg
1 recipe Egg Crêpes (p. 131)
1 recipe Creamy Parmesan Sauce (p. 135)
    (optional)

Heat a small sauté pan on medium. Add olive oil. When oil is hot but not smoking, add the garlic and sauté for 1–2 minutes or until golden brown. Place the garlic and oil in mixing bowl.

Dry spinach on a paper towel. Place it in the bowl with the ricotta and mix until well combined. Season with salt, pepper, and nutmeg.

Lay each egg crêpe flat, then place about 1/3 cup filling across the width. Roll the crêpe burrito style, and serve with the folded side down. Top with Creamy Parmesan Sauce, if desired.

Egg Crêpes with Ground Beef Filling

PRO/FATS AND VEGGIES—LEVEL ONE

MAKES 6–8 CRÊPES

2–3 tablespoons olive oil
1 onion, chopped
6 ounces mushrooms, sliced
1 pound ground beef
1/4 cup chopped fresh parsley
1 teaspoon fresh thyme (or 1/2 teaspoon dried)

1/2 teaspoon chopped fresh rosemary (or 1/4 teaspoon dried)
Salt and freshly ground black pepper
1 recipe Egg Crêpes (p. 131)
1 recipe Creamy Parmesan Sauce (p. 135) (optional)

Heat a large skillet on medium high heat. Add the olive oil, then the onion, and sauté until golden brown, about 10 minutes. Remove onions from the pan and set aside. Add a little more oil and sauté the mushrooms until browned and crusty, about 10 minutes. Set aside with the onions. Add the ground beef to the skillet with the parsley, thyme, and rosemary. Season liberally with salt and pepper. Brown until meat is cooked through. Return the onions and mushrooms to the ground beef and stir until well combined.

Lay each egg crêpe flat, then place about 1/3 cup filling across the width. Roll the crêpe burrito style, and serve with the folded side down. Top with Creamy Parmesan Sauce, if desired.

Creamy Parmesan Sauce

PRO/FATS—LEVEL ONE

MAKES ABOUT 1 1/2 CUPS

This sauce is an old standby that was big in the '70s when we all still ate fat. It went out with hot pants and bell-bottoms in the '80s when the fat-free movement swept through our nation. Thank goodness, heavy cream and cheese are back in fashion. You'll love this sauce over Egg Crêpes with any of my delicious fillings. Or pour it over a chicken breast and some broccoli for a sinful dinner.

1 cup freshly grated Parmesan cheese
½ cup heavy cream
Salt and freshly ground black pepper

Place the Parmesan in a small mixing bowl. Heat the cream in a small saucepan until it just begins to boil. Add the hot cream to the Parmesan and stir until well combined. Season with salt and pepper.

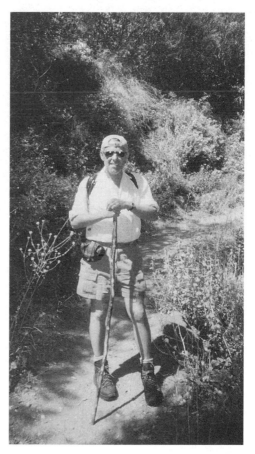

Alan, my hiking partner.

Eggs Baked in Tomatoes and Red Peppers

PRO/FATS AND VEGGIES—LEVEL ONE

SERVES 2

Alan makes me this exquisite breakfast. I'm one lucky woman.

⅛ cup extra-virgin olive oil
1 medium-size red onion, sliced
1 red bell pepper, seeded and thinly sliced
1 (28-ounce) can plum tomatoes, drained and chopped

Salt and freshly ground black pepper
4 eggs
¼ cup crumbled feta cheese

Heat a 10-inch sauté pan on medium heat. Add the oil and the onion and cook for about 5 minutes. Add the bell pepper and cook for another 7 minutes. Add the tomatoes, salt, and pepper. Reduce heat; simmer 30–40 minutes. Creating small wells in the tomato mixture, break the eggs into the tomatoes. Cover with a lid and cook until whites have set but yolks are still runny. Sprinkle with the feta cheese and serve immediately.

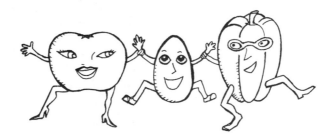

Grilled Onion Frittata

PRO/FATS AND VEGGIES—LEVEL ONE

SERVES 6

I love frittatas; they're like omelettes, but lighter and fluffier. This one is made with grilled onions and Parmesan cheese.

1 red onion, cut into 8 equal-size wedges
1 yellow onion, cut into 8 equal-size wedges
½ teaspoon salt
¼ teaspoon freshly ground black pepper
¼ cup olive oil

10 eggs
¼ cup heavy cream
½ cup freshly grated Parmesan cheese
2 tablespoons unsalted butter
1 teaspoon finely chopped fresh rosemary

Preheat oven to 350 degrees.

In a large bowl, combine onions and olive oil and toss to coat well.

Preheat a grill pan over high heat. Arrange onion wedges on grill pan and cook until browned and tender underneath, about 5 minutes. Turn onions over and cook until very tender, 5–7 minutes more. Brush with more oil as needed.

In a large bowl beat eggs and cream until blended. Stir in cheese, salt, and pepper until smooth.

In a 10-inch braiser or ovenproof frying pan over medium low heat, melt butter. Add rosemary and cook, stirring, 1 minute. Pour egg mixture into pan and fold gently to combine rosemary and eggs. Arrange grilled onions over top of eggs.

Transfer pan to oven and bake until frittata is golden brown and puffy, about 12–15 minutes.

Note

If you do not have an ovenproof frying pan, transfer the egg mixture to an 8-inch nonstick cake pan and bake as directed.

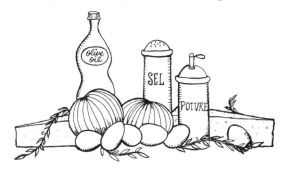

Spinach Parmesan Frittata

PRO/FATS AND VEGGIES—LEVEL ONE

SERVES 4–6

This Spinach Parmesan Frittata is the most classic version. It's great served right out of the oven, or at room temperature. When I'm having a lot of people over for brunch, this is great for a buffet. You can cook it in advance and slice it into wedges. Serve it with bacon, sausage, and a green salad. Also makes a great snack for between meals.

6 large eggs
Salt and freshly ground black pepper
Freshly grated nutmeg

4 cups loosely packed fresh spinach leaves, rinsed, dried, and finely chopped
1 cup freshly grated Parmesan cheese
1 tablespoon extra-virgin olive oil

Preheat the broiler.

Break the eggs into a large bowl and beat lightly with a fork. Add the salt and pepper, nutmeg, spinach, and half the cheese and beat lightly to combine.

In a 9-inch braiser or ovenproof nonstick skillet, heat the oil over medium heat. Add the egg mixture. Reduce the heat to low and cook unstirred for about 5 minutes. There may still be some liquid on the surface at this time. Sprinkle with the remaining cheese.

Place pan under broiler for 2 minutes or until top is puffy and golden. Remove the frittata from the broiler and let cool in the pan for 2 minutes. Invert onto a large plate or platter. Serve immediately or let the frittata cool to room temperature.

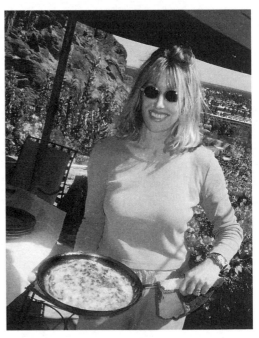

I love to make frittatas in the morning from whatever is left over in the refrigerator.

Andy's Feta and Herb Frittata

PRO/FATS AND VEGGIES—LEVEL ONE

SERVES 2

Andy was one of the amazing chefs who helped with the food for the photo shoot. One morning before the shoot, he made me this amazing frittata. One bite and I said, "Write it down! It's going in the book!"

1 medium Roma tomato
4 large eggs
1/8 teaspoon salt
Freshly ground black pepper
1 tablespoon butter

3 scallions, green part only, chopped
1 teaspoon chopped fresh rosemary
1 teaspoon chopped fresh oregano
1/3 cup plus 1/4 cup crumbled feta cheese

Preheat the broiler.

Cut the tomato crosswise. With a teaspoon scrape and remove seeds, then discard. Chop the tomato flesh into 1/2-inch pieces and set aside.

Lightly whisk the eggs in a bowl and season with salt and pepper.

In an 8-inch nonstick frying pan with an ovenproof handle, melt the butter over medium heat. Add the tomato, scallions, rosemary, and oregano. Cook and stir for 1 minute.

Remove the pan from the heat, add egg mixture to pan, and stir to evenly distribute ingredients. Lower heat, and sprinkle with feta cheese. Cook, unstirred, for 5 minutes. There may still be some liquid on the surface at this time.

Place pan under broiler for 2 minutes or until top is puffy and golden. Serve immediately.

Note

If you don't have a frying pan with an ovenproof handle, sauté the tomato, scallions, rosemary, and oregano, then mix with eggs and feta. Pour the egg mixture into an 8-inch nonstick cake pan and place in a 350 degree oven. Bake for 8–10 minutes, or until the top is puffy and golden.

Mexican Omelette

SERVES 4

I have this omelette at least once a week at a little breakfast joint in Palm Springs called The Sunshine Café. The chef is authentic Mexican, and his omelette is divine. I make mine with Lawry's Taco Seasoning! I know, I know, but it's really good. At the restaurant, they keep asking me how I can stay so thin and eat this for breakfast all the time; but we know the answer, don't we! (The Guacamole is Level Two, so if you are on Level One, eliminate this until you reach your goal weight.)

12 eggs
½ cup water
Salt and freshly ground black pepper
2 tablespoons vegetable oil (or enough to cover bottom of pan)

1 pound ground beef
1 package Lawry's taco seasoning
Sour cream for garnish
Salsa for garnish

In a medium bowl, beat the eggs and about ¼ cup water with a fork until well mixed. Add salt and pepper.

Heat a 10-inch frying pan on medium high heat. Add the vegetable oil and the ground beef. Sauté the ground beef until browned and looking minced. Add Lawry's Taco Seasoning and ¼ cup water. Turn down the heat to medium and cook until the water evaporates. Set aside.

Heat another frying pan (preferably an omelette pan) over medium to medium high heat. To make the first omelette, add a little oil and about ¼ of the beaten eggs. You don't want the pan to be too hot or the

omelette will get too brown. Let the omelette set for about 5 minutes, then, using a spatula, gently flip it over to other side. Spoon the ground beef filling on top and cook for another minute. Fold the top half over the ground beef and slide onto serving plate.

Serve immediately with a dollop of sour cream and a spoonful of salsa.

Repeat above process until all four omelettes are completed.

For Level Two
Add a spoonful of Chunky Jalapeño Guacamole (p. 150).

Drinks

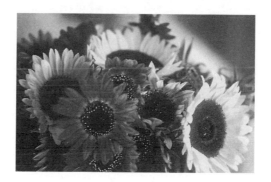

Fresh Mint Tea

SERVES 4

Everyone always asks what to drink when you're Somersizing. My pat answer is, "Water!" Now I can also say, "And my Fresh Mint Tea!" It's decaf, so you may enjoy as much as you want. And it's made with SomerSweet, which is 99.9% chemical free! Beware of chemical sweeteners!

1 cup tightly packed fresh mint leaves
4 decaffeinated tea bags
6 cups boiling water

4 sprigs fresh mint for garnish
SomerSweet or saccharin to taste

Place mint and tea bags in a glass pitcher. Pour boiling water into pitcher and let steep until room temperature. Refrigerate for at least 2 hours. Discard mint and tea bags. Place a sprig of fresh mint in the bottom of each glass. Fill the glasses with ice cubes, then pour iced tea. Sweeten with SomerSweet to your liking, or your favorite artificial sweetener.

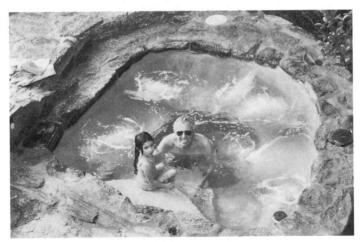

*A little R&R between courses
for Alan and his granddaughter.*

Rich Mocha Coolers

PRO/FATS—ALMOST LEVEL ONE

MAKES 2

Those frothy cappuccino drinks we've come to love at designer coffeehouses are loaded with sugar and/or chemicals. This one is made with SomerSweet, decaf coffee, and cream. It creates a minor imbalance because cocoa powder is a Funky Food (it has caffeine). If you need a little pick-me-up, this mocha cooler is the ticket.

1 cup heavy cream
½ cup freshly brewed decaffeinated coffee
½ teaspoon vanilla extract
2 tablespoons unsweetened cocoa powder

2½ teaspoons SomserSweet (or saccharin to taste)
5 ice cubes (about ½ cup)

Place cream, coffee, vanilla, cocoa powder, and SomerSweet in a blender. Blend on low speed to incorporate the ingredients. Add ice cubes and blend on high until foamy and frothy. Serve in chilled glasses.

Cool Mocha Coolers

MAKES 2

In this version I use nonfat dairy products for an Almost Level One Carbo treat.

½ cup freshly brewed decaffeinated coffee
1 cup nonfat milk
4 teaspoons nonfat dried milk powder
2½ teaspoons vanilla extract
2 tablespoons plus 2 teaspoons
    unsweetened cocoa powder

4 teaspoons SomerSweet (or saccharin to
    taste)
5 ice cubes (about ½ cup)

Place coffee, nonfat milk, nonfat powdered milk, vanilla, cocoa powder, and SomerSweet in a blender. Blend on low to incorporate all the ingredients. Add ice cubes and blend on high until light and frothy. Serve in chilled glasses.

Sauces, Dips, and Dressings

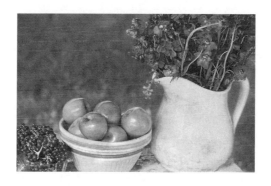

Blue Cheese Dip

PRO/FATS—LEVEL ONE

MAKES ABOUT 1 1/2 CUPS

This dip is a winner with chopped celery sticks and my delicious Buffalo Wings. Can you believe you're losing weight eating this?

3/4 cup sour cream
4 ounces crumbled blue cheese (I like
    Maytag Blue and Roquefort)

2 tablespoons red wine vinegar
Salt
Freshly ground black pepper

Combine all ingredients in a bowl, mashing the cheese with a fork until well combined. If the dressing is too thick, add a little more vinegar.

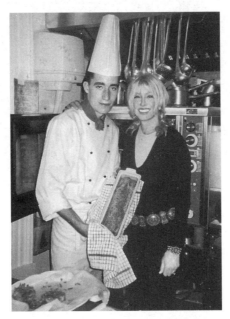

A cooking lesson from the chef at
St. Clerins, Merv Griffin's house in Ireland.

Hot Crab Dip

PRO/FATS AND VEGGIES—LEVEL ONE

MAKES ABOUT 1 1/2 CUPS

This recipe has been around forever. Traditionally it's served with crackers. To make it Somersized, I serve it with Parmesan Chips (p. 170) and crudités. You can even cut the tops off little cherry tomatoes, hollow them out, and stuff the dip inside.

2 (6-ounce) cans crabmeat
4 ounces cream cheese, softened
1/2 cup mayonnaise
1/4 cup freshly grated Parmesan cheese

2 scallions, finely chopped
1/2 teaspoon salt
1/2 teaspoon prepared horseradish

Mix all the ingredients for the dip in a glass or microwave safe bowl. Heat for 1–2 minutes or until nice and hot.

Serving Suggestion
Serve with Parmesan Chips (p. 170) or with crudités such as cherry tomatoes or celery, zucchini, or jicama sticks.

Spinach Dip

MAKES 3 1/2 CUPS

This traditional dip is usually served in a hollowed-out sourdough bread "bowl." You can't have the bread, but you can still enjoy this timeless favorite. Serve it with your favorite Somersize vegetable sticks.

1 (16-ounce) bag frozen chopped spinach,
    thawed and dried
1 cup mayonnaise
1/2 cup sour cream
1 stalk celery, finely chopped
1 (6-ounce) can water chestnuts, drained
    and finely chopped

1/2 teaspoon lemon juice
1/8 teaspoon nutmeg
1/8 teaspoon cayenne pepper
Salt and freshly ground black pepper
    to taste

After thawing the spinach, place it in a salad spinner to dry it. (Or place it in a clean dish towel and squeeze out the liquid.) Mix all the ingredients for the dip together. Chill an hour before serving.

Serving Suggestion
Serve with a crudité platter of jicama sticks, celery sticks, and drained hearts of palm.

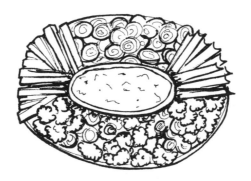

Green Goddess Dressing

MAKES ABOUT 1½ CUPS

This is one of those "I can't believe I can eat this and still lose weight" dressings. No fat-free, tasteless, bottled dressing on this program. Use it as a dip with artichokes, as a dressing with Southern Country Fried Chicken Salad (p.178), and as a sauce for Crispy Fried Catfish (p. 212). Divine!

4 scallions
1½ cups mayonnaise

Juice from 2 limes (about ¼ cup)

Trim the ends off the scallions. Roughly chop the white and green parts and place in a food processor or blender. Chop until coarsely ground. Add the mayonnaise and lime juice, and puree until smooth. Dressing will store in the refrigerator for a week or more in a sealed container.

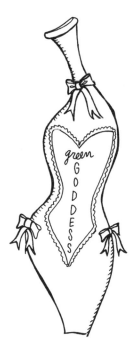

Chunky Jalapeño Guacamole

LEVEL TWO

MAKES ABOUT 2 CUPS

Guacamole is made with avocado, a Funky Food that has fat and carbohydrate. However, it is a welcome addition on Level Two and particularly great on my Mexican Omelette (p.140). It's also great spread on whole-grain bread and piled with vegetables for a Level Two sandwich.

2 large ripe avocados, peeled and pitted
2 Roma tomatoes, diced
3 tablespoons finely chopped red onion
2 tablespoons finely chopped cilantro

1 tablespoon lime juice
2 teaspoons finely minced jalapeño pepper
Salt and freshly ground black pepper

Mash avocados with a fork in a large bowl until chunky. Mix in tomatoes. Add the remaining ingredients. Season with salt and pepper. Can be made up to 3 hours ahead. For storage, press plastic wrap onto surface of guacamole and chill.

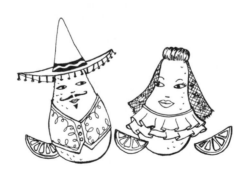

Salsa de Perez

VEGGIES—LEVEL ONE

MAKES ABOUT 4 CUPS

Ripe tomatoes, crunchy radishes, spicy jalapeños. Pair this salsa with Carne Asada de Perez (p. 245) for a knockout Pro/Fats and Veggies meal, or with Black Bean Vegetable Chili (p. 204) for a great Carbos and Veggies meal.

3 large tomatoes, seeded and chopped
2 bunches cilantro, chopped
1 cup chopped onion
4 jalapeño peppers, seeded and finely
   chopped

1 bunch radishes, chopped
2 cups freshly squeezed lemon juice
Salt

The key to this recipe is chopping all the vegetables about the same size. Then gently toss all the ingredients to combine. Salt to taste and set aside for at least 1 hour to let the flavors combine.

(Don't put your salsa in the refrigerator or the tomatoes will get mushy. However, if you have leftovers you'll want to refrigerate it overnight to keep for the next day.)

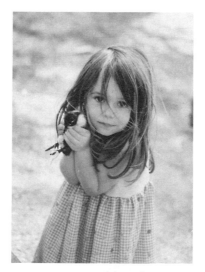

My granddaughter.

Lemon Tarragon Vinaigrette

PRO/FATS—LEVEL ONE

MAKES 1 CUP

My mother used a lot of tarragon in her cooking. I love this lemony tarragon dressing. It's made with lemon juice and lemon zest. Zest is the colored outer skin or peel. A vegetable peeler or citrus zester will remove this flavorful peel without touching the white pith, which is bitter.

½ cup tarragon vinegar
½ teaspoon chopped fresh thyme
1 teaspoon chopped fresh oregano
1 teaspoon freshly squeezed lemon juice

½ teaspoon grated lemon zest
⅓ cup extra-virgin olive oil
¼ teaspoon salt
⅛ teaspoon freshly ground black pepper

In a small bowl, whisk the vinegar, herbs, lemon juice, and zest. Gradually whisk in the olive oil. As it combines or emulsifies, the dressing will start to thicken. Season with salt and pepper, then taste and adjust seasonings. Store in the refrigerator in a sealed container. Dressing will last a week or more.

Red Wine Vinaigrette

PRO/FATS—LEVEL ONE

MAKES ABOUT 1 CUP

This tangy salad dressing will last in the refrigerator for about a week. Store it in a screw-top jar and give it a shake just before use.

½ cup red wine vinegar
½ teaspoon dried oregano
½ teaspoon lemon juice

⅓ cup extra-virgin olive oil
⅛ teaspoon salt
⅛ teaspoon freshly ground black pepper

Mix vinegar, oregano, and lemon juice in a blender (or whisk by hand). With blender running (or whisking constantly), slowly drizzle in the olive oil. Your dressing will thicken and emulsify. Add salt and pepper to taste.

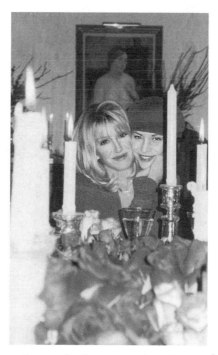

Me and my darling stepdaughter, Leslie.

Artichoke Pesto

PRO/FATS AND VEGGIES—LEVEL ONE

MAKES ABOUT 3 CUPS

This pesto is delicious served as a cold dip with crudités (cut-up vegetables). For Level Two, try it with whole wheat pita triangles, or sauté it and toss with whole wheat pasta and vegetables.

2 (14-ounce) cans artichoke bottoms,
   drained
6 cloves garlic, chopped
1/2 cup mayonnaise
1/2 cup freshly grated Parmesan cheese

4 scallions, chopped
2 teaspoons freshly squeezed lemon juice
1/2 cup olive oil
Salt and freshly ground black pepper

Place all ingredients in a food processor and pulse until smooth. Season with salt and pepper to taste.

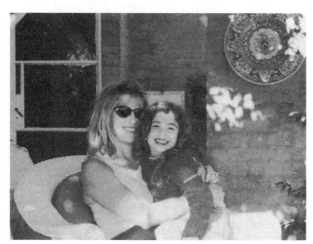

I love my grandchildren!

Basil Pesto

MAKES ABOUT 1 1/2 CUPS

Pesto is a staple in every Italian kitchen. I am never without it in my refrigerator. When I come home from a long trip, I always know I have a Level Two meal in the house if there's pasta in the pantry and a jar of pesto.

There are many, many ways to use pesto. Serve it over fresh tomatoes and buffalo mozzarella. A dollop of pesto is great on your favorite soup. Or try it as a topping for chicken or lamb. Pesto also makes a great roasted chicken. Rub the pesto underneath the skin of the chicken so that the pesto is between the skin and the breast meat. Then rub the outside of the chicken with additional pesto before baking.

1 or more cloves garlic
3 tablespoons unsalted butter
1/4 teaspoon ground white pepper
Pinch of freshly grated nutmeg
1/2 cup freshly grated Parmesan cheese

2 cups loosely packed basil leaves, stems removed
1/4 cup Italian parsley leaves, stems removed
1/4 cup extra-virgin olive oil
Salt and freshly ground black pepper

To a food processor fitted with the steel blade, add the garlic, butter, white pepper, and nutmeg. With the food processor running, add the Parmesan, then the basil and the parsley. Trickle the oil into the processor until the sauce is smooth. If necessary, add a little hot water to the sauce in order to reach the desired consistency. Then add salt and pepper to taste.

For Level Two
To the garlic, butter, pepper, and nutmeg, add 2 tablespoons walnuts and 1 tablespoon pine nuts. Prepare as above and toss with some whole-grain pasta.

Sun-Dried Tomato Pesto

PRO/FATS AND VEGGIES—LEVEL ONE

MAKES 1 1/2 CUPS

Sun-dried tomatoes came about as a result of the tomato harvest in Italy, when they are in such abundance that in order for the tomatoes not to go bad, the farmers slice them, lay them out on baking sheets, and let them dry in the sun. Now we can do the same thing in the oven. You will find many uses for this delicious pesto. It serves as a dip for vegetables, or for Level Two, toss it with whole wheat pasta or spread it on grilled bread.

12 tomatoes, thinly sliced
Sea salt

Freshly ground black pepper
1/4 cup extra-virgin olive oil

Preheat the oven to its lowest temperature—about 150 degrees.

Lay the tomato slices on baking sheets. Sprinkle them with salt and pepper and a little olive oil. Place in the center of oven. Let the tomatoes dry for about 3 hours. They should feel dry to the touch but not dried out. A little bit of wetness keeps the flavor really nice. Rotate the baking sheets every now and then so the tomatoes cook evenly.

Remove tomatoes from oven and put them, in batches, into your food processor. Pulse until roughly pureed. Store in the refrigerator.

Red Wine Butter Sauce

MAKES 2 CUPS

This red wine sauce brings fish, poultry, or meat to life. Try it with my Orange Roughy with Mushroom Stuffing (p. 215). When it comes to cooking wine, it should be good enough to drink. Bad wine makes bad sauce.

4 shallots, chopped
½ cup red wine
½ cup red wine vinegar

4 tablespoons heavy cream
1 pound butter, cut into 1-inch cubes
Salt and freshly ground black pepper

Combine shallots, wine, and vinegar in a saucepan. Bring to a boil, then reduce heat and simmer until almost all the liquid has evaporated and becomes thick and syrupy. Add heavy cream and mix well. Increase heat to high, but don't let the sauce boil. Add the butter and continue to whisk until all the butter is incorporated. Season with salt and pepper.

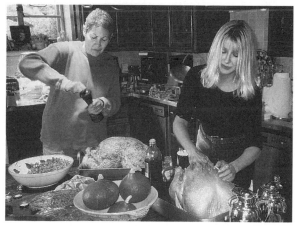

My sister-in-law Cecile and me preparing Thanksgiving dinner.

Roasted Turkey Gravy

PRO/FATS AND VEGGIES—LEVEL ONE

MAKES ABOUT 1 CUP

If you are deep-frying your turkey (which I highly recommend), you won't have any pan drippings to make gravy. In this recipe I roast wings and drumsticks to get the drippings for gravy. I suggest making this the day before; then you will not have to contend with last-minute gravy making.

8 to 10 turkey wings
4 turkey drumsticks
¼ cup olive oil
6 onions, quartered
3 parsnips, scrubbed and quartered
  (see Note)
2 cloves garlic

4 stalks celery, quartered
2 tomatoes, halved
2 tablespoons fresh thyme
Salt and freshly ground black pepper
2 quarts chicken or turkey stock
4 tablespoons butter

Preheat oven to 350 degrees.

Arrange the turkey pieces in a large roasting pan. Rub them with oil. Add the rest of the ingredients except the stock and the butter. Season liberally with salt and pepper.

Roast in 350 degree oven for 1½ hours. Remove the turkey pieces and reserve for another meal. Discard the vegetables. Turn burner heat to high and place roasting pan with drippings on it. When drippings are bubbling, begin to add stock, 2 cups at a time. Constantly scrape the bits from bottom of roasting pan. As the stock reduces, add another 2 cups until all the stock is incorporated.

Your gravy will turn a rich golden brown and reduce to a syrupy consistency. Taste for seasonings. Turn heat off and stir in the 4 tablespoons of butter.

Serve immediately, and pass extra in a gravy boat.

Note

Parsnips create a minor imbalance. If you are doing well on Level One, you should not have a problem incorporating them.

Soups

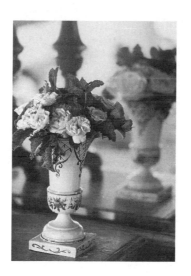

Cream of Green Chili Soup

SERVES 4

Rich, spicy, creamy, and easy. Just the way I like my soup. For an extra kick of heat you can add a chipotle chili (a dried, smoked jalapeño chili), available in most markets. If you can't find it, the soup is still delicious without it.

1 (4-ounce) can whole peeled green chilies
1 chipotle chili (optional)
1 (14.5-ounce) can chicken broth

4 ounces cream cheese
⅓ cup heavy cream
Salt and freshly ground black pepper

Put all ingredients in a blender or food processor and puree until smooth. Heat in a saucepan and serve immediately.

Quick Chicken Broth

PRO/FATS AND VEGGIES—LEVEL ONE

SERVES 6–8

Broth is one of the most important staples in my kitchen. I like this one because it's fast and flavorful.

3 pounds chicken, quartered (include all
   giblets)
1 (10½-ounce) can beef broth
2 onions, quartered
3 stalks celery, cut into chunks
1 parsnip, scrubbed and quartered
   (see Note)

1 parsley root (optional)
1 large bunch fresh parsley, chopped
2 bunches fresh dill
1 tablespoon coarse salt

Put the chicken and giblets into a large pot. Add the beef broth and enough water to just cover the chicken. Bring to a boil. Skim off the fat.

Add the onions, celery, parsnip, optional parsley root, parsley, dill, and salt. Cover and simmer for 1½ hours. Skim off the fat.

Strain the broth into a clean pot. Peel off the usable meat from the chicken pieces and reserve for use in your favorite soup or chicken salad. Discard the bones and veg-etables. Store the clear broth in plastic con-tainers in the freezer, until ready to use. Or store the broth in plastic bags and lay them flat in the freezer. Makes defrosting in the microwave a cinch.

Note
Parsnips are technically a Funky Food, but if you are doing well on Level One, you should not have a problem adding this small amount to this broth.

Egg Crêpe Noodles in Chicken Broth

PRO/FATS AND VEGGIES—LEVEL ONE

SERVES 4

My mother-in-law, Margaret, made the best chicken soup with beautiful egg crêpe noodles. I loved her dearly, and I loved her soup. This is comfort food of the highest order.

4–6 Egg Crêpes (p. 131)
4 cups Quick Chicken Broth (p. 161)
  or canned chicken broth

Salt and freshly ground black pepper
½ cup chopped fresh parsley

To make the egg crêpes into noodles, roll each crêpe, then slice into noodles approximately ½ inch wide. If they are too narrow, they tend to disintegrate in the hot soup.

Fill bowls with hot broth and add a handful of noodles just before you serve. Season to taste with salt and freshly ground pepper. Garnish with fresh parsley.

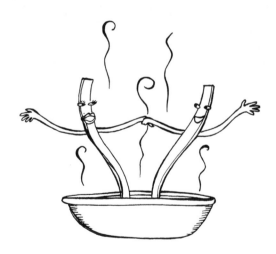

Chicken Meatball Asparagus Soup

SERVES 4

My incomparable housekeeper, Shanthi, also happens to be a phenomenal cook. Alan and I had just come home from a long trip and Shanthi had two big bowls of this delicious soup waiting for us. It's a totally filling and satisfying meal. I've probably requested it twenty-five times since she made it the first time! After word of her soup gets out, she'll be writing cookbooks!

10 tablespoons olive oil
1 medium onion, chopped
1 large bunch asparagus, thinly sliced,
    washed and tough lower stems removed
5 leeks, white part only, thinly sliced

6 cups fresh or canned chicken broth
1 pound ground chicken
Salt and freshly ground black pepper

Heat a stockpot over medium high heat. Add 3 tablespoons olive oil. Add the onion and sauté until light brown, about 7–10 minutes. Add asparagus and leeks. Sauté another 5 minutes. Add the chicken broth and bring to a boil, then reduce heat and simmer for about 15 minutes.

Meanwhile, mix the ground chicken with salt and pepper. Make small meatballs, about 1 inch in diameter. In a 10-inch skillet, heat 6–7 tablespoons of olive oil and fry the meatballs until brown on all sides. Add the meatballs to the soup.

Roasted Sweet Red Pepper Soup with Crème Fraîche and Crispy Sage Leaves

PRO/FATS AND VEGGIES—LEVEL ONE

SERVES 6–8

I love this soup. It's rich and roasted, beautiful and professional-looking, but you will be amazed at how easy it is to prepare. I first tasted this soup in Tuscany at the home of my dear friend Marco Montanari. He drizzled olive oil in his bowl right before serving, but I added crème fraîche and loved what it did to the flavor. Try it both ways and decide. For my Southwest Christmas dinner, this soup looked so beautiful and festive. A little goes a long way, so be sure to serve it in small bowls if it is a first course.

2 tablespoons extra-virgin olive oil
1 stalk celery, minced
1 onion, minced
6 red bell peppers, roasted and sliced
   (p. 165)
Salt to taste

1 medium-size celery root, diced
1 quart water
2 cups Quick Chicken Broth (p. 161)
   or canned chicken broth
¼ cup crème fraîche or sour cream
Fried Sage Leaves for garnish (p. 165)

In a large stockpot, combine olive oil, celery, and onion. Cook over moderate heat until the vegetables are soft and fragrant, about 10 to 15 minutes. Add the sliced roasted peppers and cook 3 to 4 minutes more for greater flavor intensity. Season with salt. Add celery root, water, and chicken broth. Cover and cook over moderate heat until the celery root is soft, about 40 minutes.

Puree with a hand mixer or transfer in batches to a blender or food processor. Serve in warm shallow soup bowls. Drizzle each bowl with crème fraîche or sour cream in an attractive pattern.

Sprinkle a few fried sage leaves on top for garnish and flavor.

Fried Sage Leaves

Enough olive oil to cover bottom of pan
40 fresh sage leaves, washed and patted dry

Salt

Heat a skillet on medium heat. Add the olive oil. When oil is hot but not smoking, add sage leaves. Fry till crispy. Drain on paper towels. Sprinkle with salt. Save until ready to use as garnish.

Roasted Peppers
VEGGIES—LEVEL ONE

Roasted peppers make everything taste great. They're easy to prepare with this simple technique. Serve them with grilled bread for a Carbos and Veggies meal or with any of your favorite salads, poultry, meat, or fish for a hearty Pro/Fats and Veggies meal. Or puree them in my wonderful Roasted Sweet Red Pepper Soup with Crème Fraîche and Crispy Sage Leaves (p. 164).

Your favorite peppers

Place the whole peppers on a prepared hot grill or an open flame on the stove and char on all sides until the skins are black and bubbling. Immediately put the roasted peppers into a plastic bag and seal. Let the peppers steam in the bag for about 15 minutes. (This steaming process will make the peeling easier.)

Remove the peppers from the bag and pull the stems off. Break the peppers apart and discard the seeds. The charred skin will peel off easily. I find it's faster to seed and peel the peppers under cool running water. Break into strips and use as needed.

Stracciatella Soup

SERVES 6

This easy-to-prepare Tuscan soup is truly satisfying. In Italian, stracciatelle means "little rags" or "strings," which is what the eggs look like when they are dropped into the soup and then cooked. After a long day, this soup really hits the spot.

4 cups Quick Chicken Broth (p. 161)
   or canned chicken broth
6 ounces spinach, fresh, or frozen, thawed,
   and drained

2 eggs, lightly beaten
Salt and freshly ground black pepper
   to taste
1/4 cup freshly grated Parmesan cheese

Bring chicken broth to a boil. Add spinach and simmer for about 4 minutes. Quickly stir in beaten eggs, and continue to stir vigorously until eggs have coagulated and turned white.

Ladle into soup bowls, and season with salt and pepper. Spoon Parmesan cheese on top. Serve immediately.

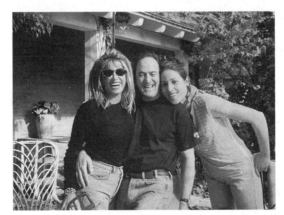

Good friends. Marco and Sandra from Tuscany visiting us in the desert.

Watercress Mushroom Soup

PRO/FATS AND VEGGIES—LEVEL ONE

SERVES 4–6

This recipe yields 4–6 servings, unless my son Bruce is at the table. He loves this soup! Every time I make it for him he says, "Ma, this is my favorite soup." Of all my careers, being a mother has been the most rewarding.

3 tablespoons butter
8 ounces fresh mushrooms, chopped
1 large onion, chopped
2 bunches watercress, chopped

2 cloves garlic, chopped
2 (14.5-ounce) cans chicken broth
Salt and freshly ground black pepper
5 tablespoons heavy cream

Heat a large sauté pan on medium heat. Add the butter. When butter is melted, add the mushrooms and onion. Sauté about 5 minutes. Add the chopped watercress and garlic and sauté for another 10 minutes. Stir in 1 can of chicken broth.

Puree the mixture using a hand mixer or by transferring to a blender or food processor.

Return the mixture to a saucepan and add rest of the broth, salt, and pepper. Stir in the cream just before serving.

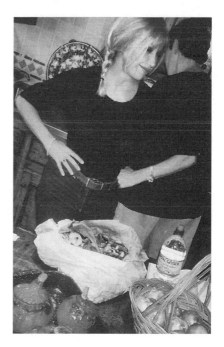

So far it looks good! Wild mushrooms, fresh onions. Could be the beginning of a great stuffing or soup!

Salads

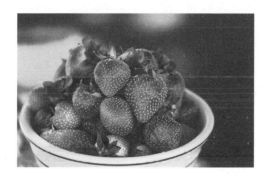

Parmesan Chips

PRO/FATS AND VEGGIES—LEVEL ONE

MAKES 24 CHIPS

I'm always looking for great bread substitutes. These Parmesan chips really hit the spot. They make delicious little chips or crackers to serve with dip, to garnish a salad or soup, or to munch all on their own. I love them with a sun-dried tomato on top. The secret to these delicious and easy chips is an 8-inch nonstick pan and using shredded, not grated, Parmesan. Use the small shredder on your grater, or buy preshredded Parmesan.

½ cup freshly shredded Parmesan cheese

Heat an 8-inch nonstick sauté pan over low to medium heat.

Sprinkle half the cheese evenly in the pan, making a circle or "pancake." Leave "pancake" 2–3 minutes until melted, and flip with a spatula. Brown the second side.

Remove from pan to a cutting board. While still warm, cut the "pancake" like a pizza into 12 triangular chips (a pizza cutter or sharp knife works great).

Repeat with remaining cheese.

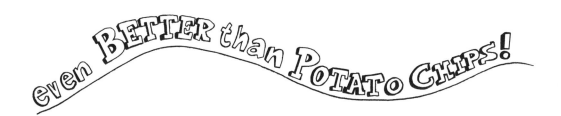

even BETTER than POTATO CHIPS!

Parmesan Croutons

PRO/FATS AND VEGGIES—LEVEL ONE

MAKES ABOUT 8 CROUTONS

If you miss the croutons in your favorite salad or soup, you'll love these Parmesan Croutons. They're just like my Parmesan Chips, but made into little squares. Use an 8-inch nonstick pan and shredded, not grated, Parmesan for best results.

½ cup freshly shredded Parmesan cheese

Heat pan over low to medium heat.

Sprinkle cheese evenly in the pan, making a circle or "pancake." Leave "pancake" 2–3 minutes until melted, and flip with a spatula. Brown the second side.

While the "pancake" is still warm, wrap it around the handle of a wooden spoon, rolling the handle to make a log. Remove the handle of the spoon and flatten the log with your hand. Cut into 1-inch squares.

Repeat with remaining cheese.

Parmesan Bowls with Caesar Salad
PRO/FATS AND VEGGIES—LEVEL ONE

MAKES 1 BOWL

Parmesan bowls are not only beautiful but edible as well. You will love the taste of these delicious salty, cheesy, chewy bowls. These make up for not having bread or rolls with your salad. Frankly, I think you will find, as I have, that you will like these better. It is essential to use a nonstick skillet (such as Teflon) and to be sure the pan is hot but not too hot. Also, I find that shredded Parmesan works better than grated Parmesan.

1½ cups freshly shredded Parmesan cheese

1 recipe Caesar Salad (p. 173)

To make the Parmesan Bowls you must have 4 small soup bowls or 4 small "jelly jar" style glasses standing by. Turn the soup bowls or glasses upside-down on the counter.

Heat an 8-inch nonstick skillet on medium.

Sprinkle shredded Parmesan cheese into the skillet and quickly spread it around until it is evenly dispersed over the entire pan.

When cheese starts to bubble, about 3 minutes, gently lift with a nonstick spatula and turn over to brown on the other side, another 2–3 minutes. When both sides are golden, slide the cheese "pancake" out of pan and onto the upside-down soup bowl or glass. Gently press cheese to conform to the shape of the soup bowl or glass. Let sit for a few minutes, until ready to serve with salad inside.

Caesar Salad

SERVES 4

This is my famous Caesar recipe from Eat Great, Lose Weight. *I'm including it again because I now have my delicious Parmesan Croutons (p. 171) to add. Or for a spectacular presentation, serve it in my Parmesan Bowls (p. 172).*

1 head romaine lettuce, rinsed and dried
Caesar Dressing (recipe follows)
1 recipe Parmesan Croutons (p. 171)

1 lemon, quartered, for garnish
Salt and freshly ground black pepper

Tear the lettuce into small pieces and toss with dressing and Parmesan Croutons.

Garnish with lemon wedges. Season with salt and pepper.

Caesar Dressing

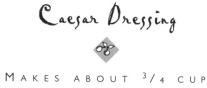

MAKES ABOUT ³/₄ CUP

I'm not an anchovy person, but if you like them, feel free to add a few mashed up in the dressing. Or use anchovy paste.

1 egg
Juice from 1 lemon
Dash of Tabasco or other hot sauce
4 mashed anchovies (or 1 tablespoon
    anchovy paste) (optional)

Salt and freshly ground black pepper
¹/₂ cup extra-virgin olive oil
¹/₂ cup freshly grated Parmesan cheese

Coddle the egg by boiling it in a saucepan for 20 seconds. Using a slotted spoon, remove the egg, crack it, and scoop out the inside into a medium bowl. Add the lemon juice, Tabasco, optional anchovies, salt, and pepper. Mix with fork until well combined. Add the olive oil in a slow stream, stirring constantly. Finish by adding the cheese. Adjust seasonings to taste.

Arugula and Parmesan Salad

PRO/FATS AND VEGGIES—LEVEL ONE

SERVES 4

I call Alan's daughter, Leslie, "the hippest chick I know." She's my clothing designer and I love her dearly. We spend a lot of time together discussing designs and having fittings at the tailor. Right near the tailor there's a fabulous little sidewalk café that serves the best Italian food. Leslie and I have shared many laughs over this salad, which I have duplicated here. It has toasted pine nuts, which are a little treat to save for Level Two.

½ cup pine nuts (only for Level Two)
1 pound arugula leaves, stems removed (or fresh baby spinach leaves)
One 2-ounce chunk Parmesan cheese

About 4 tablespoons extra-virgin olive oil
About 2 tablespoons red wine vinegar
Salt and freshly ground black pepper

Preheat the oven to 350 degrees.

Spread the nuts loosely on a baking sheet. Toast until lightly browned, 8 to 10 minutes. Check every few minutes to avoid burning the nuts. Remove from the oven and turn out onto a large plate to cool. (The nuts can be toasted several hours in advance.)

In a large shallow salad bowl, combine the arugula and toasted pine nuts. Using a vegetable peeler, shave the Parmesan cheese into long thick strips directly into the bowl. (When the chunk of cheese becomes too small to peel, grate the remaining cheese and add to the bowl.)

Drizzle the olive oil and vinegar over the salad and toss. Season with salt and pepper to taste.

Serve immediately.

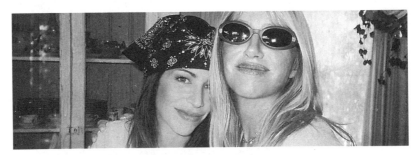

Dear Leslie and me.

Israeli Salad

VEGGIES—LEVEL ONE

SERVES 6

My friend Tuvia was born in Israel and loves all the good things in life. One summer weekend, while he and his wife, Kristi, were visiting our beach home, he made this salad, and now it is a favorite. Kirby or Persian cucumbers are the small little pickling cucumbers. They have a great flavor, but if you can't find them, you can substitute regular cucumbers. For a Carbos and Veggies meal, serve with grilled crusty multigrain bread. For a Pro/Fats and Veggies meal, add a great-quality extra-virgin olive oil. If you have the oil and the bread, it becomes Level Two.

6–7 Kirby or Persian cucumbers (or 1 regular cucumber)
4–5 tomatoes, seeded
1 green bell pepper, seeded

3 scallions
4 radishes
Salt and freshly ground black pepper

Finely dice all the vegetables into a uniform size. Toss with salt and pepper. Serve immediately or refrigerate until ready to serve.

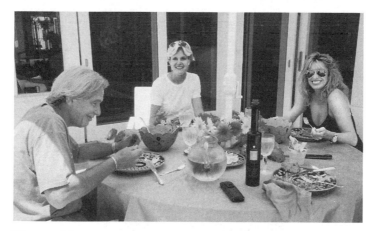

This is Tuvia, who gave me the recipe for Israeli Salad.
His wife, Kristi, did all the chopping.

Hearts of Palm and Green Bean Salad

PRO/FATS AND VEGGIES—LEVEL ONE

SERVES 4

This is a great salad for entertaining. It can be prepared and dressed and chilled several hours before guests arrive. Add the tomatoes right before serving because tomatoes get mushy when you refrigerate them.

Salt
1 pound green beans
1 (14.5-ounce) can hearts of palm, drained
2 medium Roma tomatoes, seeded and
 chopped

2 red onions, thinly sliced
1 bunch Italian parsley, chopped
2 ounces feta cheese, crumbled
1 recipe Red Wine Vinaigrette (p. 153)
Freshly ground black pepper

Bring a saucepan of salted water to a boil. Add the green beans and boil about 3–4 minutes, until tender. The beans will change from light to dark green. Drain and plunge the beans into a bowl of ice water. The ice bath stops the cooking process, sets the flavor, and helps the beans retain their dark green color. Slice the blanched green beans on the diagonal into 1-inch pieces and place in a large bowl.

Slice the hearts of palm on the diagonal into 1-inch pieces. Add the hearts of palm, tomatoes, onions, parsley, and feta cheese to the green beans. Toss with the Red Wine Vinaigrette. Season with additional salt and freshly ground pepper.

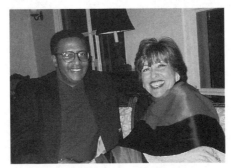

Our friends Andrea and Nelson are frequent dinner guests at our home.

Salad à la Niçoise

SERVES 2

This traditional French salad from Nice is made with tuna, green beans, hard-boiled egg, and pota-toes. I substituted celery root for the potatoes and, "Voilà!" it's Somersized. This salad tastes great made with fresh ahi tuna or with a 12-ounce can of albacore tuna packed in water. Just drain the tuna and flake it with fresh lemon juice, salt, and pepper.

2–4 ounces fresh ahi tuna fillets
Salt and freshly ground black pepper
1 tablespoon olive oil
2 cloves garlic, sliced thick
1 small red onion, sliced in rings
8 ounces green beans, trimmed and
    steamed

1 small celery root, cubed and steamed
1 recipe Lemon Tarragon Vinaigrette
    (p. 152)
1 Roma tomato, cut in 4 wedges
2 hard-boiled eggs, sliced in half
2 tablespoons finely chopped fresh parsley

Season the tuna fillets with salt and pep-per. Heat the oil in a sauté pan. Add the garlic. Brown the garlic for 2–3 minutes, then add the tuna. Cook the fillets for 3–4 minutes on each side. Remove fillets and garlic from pan and reserve in warm oven. Add the onion rings in the pan, stirring until they wilt.

Toss the steamed green beans and celery root in about 2 tablespoons of the vinai-grette. Arrange the dressed beans in the center of the plate, with celery root on either side. Place the tuna and garlic on the green beans. Drizzle with dressing. Mound the red onions on top of the tuna. Arrange tomato wedges and hard-boiled eggs on the side. Sprinkle with chopped parsley.

Southern Country Fried Chicken Salad

PRO/FATS AND VEGGIES—LEVEL ONE

SERVES 2

Bruce and Caroline spent a week with us last summer to hang out at our beach house with the kids. We had such fun playing on the beach and collecting seashells with the girls. As an added bonus, Caroline made this delicious salad for lunch with my fabulous Green Goddess Dressing. It's heaven-sent!

1 head romaine lettuce, washed and
   chopped
2 cucumbers, peeled and sliced
3 stalks celery, chopped
2–3 cups peanut oil

4 boneless, skinless chicken breasts,
   chopped into 1-inch cubes
Salt and freshly ground black pepper
1 recipe Green Goddess Dressing (p. 149)
1 pint basket cherry tomatoes

Place the lettuce in a large bowl. Add the cucumbers and celery.

Heat the oil in a deep skillet on medium high heat. Season the chicken pieces with salt and pepper. Add the chicken to the hot oil and fry for about 5 minutes, until golden brown. Drain on paper towels.

Toss the lettuce with about ¾ cup of the dressing. (You can store the additional dressing in the refrigerator.) Top with the chicken pieces and garnish with cherry tomatoes. Serve immediately.

For Level Two
Add a sprinkle of corn and toasted pecans.

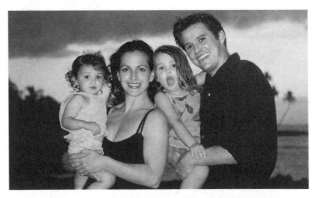

*My son, Bruce, and his beautiful family—
his wife, Caroline, and darling daughters.*

Red Bean and Parsley Salad

I love these red beans with a big salad for lunch. Alan and I sit on the deck at the beach and enjoy this simple summer meal as we watch the waves crash onto the sand. It's also great at room temperature for a buffet spread or a picnic. At parties I always like to give Pro/Fats and Carbos options so that everyone can choose what they like.

2½ cups (1 pound) dried red beans
1 onion, halved
3 bay leaves
4 cloves garlic, crushed
1 stalk celery, chopped into 2 pieces
1 sprig fresh sage

6 tablespoons extra-virgin olive oil
1 red onion, finely chopped
¼ cup red wine vinegar
Salt and freshly ground black pepper
1 bunch Italian parsley leaves, chopped

Rinse the beans, picking them over to remove any debris. Place beans in a large bowl with enough water to cover by 2 inches. Let soak overnight. For a faster soak, add boiling water to cover and set aside for 1 hour. Drain the beans, discarding the water.

Place the onion, bay leaves, garlic, celery, sage, and 2 tablespoons of the oil in a large saucepan and add cold water to cover by 1 inch. Cover pan and bring to a boil over moderate heat, then reduce to a simmer and cook for 15 minutes. Add the drained beans and return to a boil. Reduce heat and cover beans, cooking until tender, about 45 minutes. The beans are done when they are still slightly firm but not mushy.

Meanwhile, in a small bowl, toss the chopped onions with 2 tablespoons of the oil. Set aside.

Once the beans are cooked, drain them, discarding the herbs and vegetables. Transfer the beans to a large bowl. While still warm, toss with the chopped onion and the remaining 2 tablespoons of oil, the vinegar, salt, and pepper. Serve immediately or reserve in the refrigerator. Bring to room temperature before serving, or reheat in a skillet.

Salads
179

White Bean Salad with Sage and Thyme

LEVEL TWO

SERVES 8–10

I became a big fan of white beans after traveling in Tuscany. This salad can be served warm or at room temperature. It makes a healthy and delicious Level Two lunch served with fresh tomatoes and grilled whole-grain bread.

1½ cups (1 pound) dried small white beans
   (navy, cannellini, or toscanelli)
1 yellow onion, halved
3 bay leaves
4 cloves garlic, crushed
1 stalk celery, chopped into 2 pieces
1 sprig fresh sage (or 1 teaspoon dried)

1 sprig fresh thyme (or 1 teaspoon
   dried)
½ cup extra-virgin olive oil
3 tablespoons chopped fresh thyme leaves
   (or 1½ teaspoons dried thyme)
1 red onion, finely chopped
Salt and freshly ground black pepper

Rinse the beans, picking them over to remove any debris. Place beans in a large bowl with enough water to cover by 2 inches. Let soak overnight. For a faster soak, add boiling water to cover and set aside for 1 hour. Drain the beans, discarding the water.

Place the drained beans in a large saucepan and add cold water to cover by 1 inch. Add the onion, bay leaves, garlic, celery, sage and thyme sprigs, and 2 tablespoons of the oil. Cover and bring to a boil over medium heat, then reduce and simmer for about 1 hour. Add more water if the liquid is drying out. The beans are done when they are still slightly firm but not mushy.

Drain the cooked beans and discard the vegetables and herb sprigs. Transfer the beans to a large bowl. While still warm, toss with the chopped thyme and chopped red onion. Season with salt and pepper and add the remaining 6 tablespoons olive oil. Serve immediately or reserve in the refrigerator. Bring to room temperature before serving, or reheat in a skillet.

Bread and Pasta

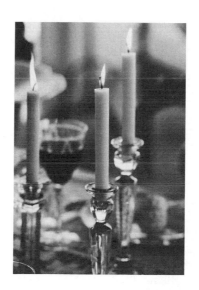

Whole Wheat Bread

CARBOS—LEVEL ONE

MAKES 1 (1½-POUND) LOAF

I've received so many letters asking for bread recipes. Now we have it! You'll need an automatic bread machine, available at cooking stores. Have a couple of slices in the morning with nonfat cottage cheese and a sprinkle of cinnamon. Whole wheat bread flour is best because of the high gluten content. If you can't find it, use whole wheat pastry flour.

5 cups whole wheat bread flour
2 teaspoons salt
2 cups water

⅔ cup nonfat dried milk powder
½ cup nonfat plain yogurt
1 tablespoon active dry yeast

Mix together whole wheat bread flour and salt in a bowl. Set aside.

In a saucepan whisk together water and milk powder. Stir in the nonfat yogurt. Using an instant-read thermometer, heat the mixture to 80 degrees over low heat.

Place all the ingredients in a bread machine following the manufacturer's guidelines. Bake using the whole wheat cycle.

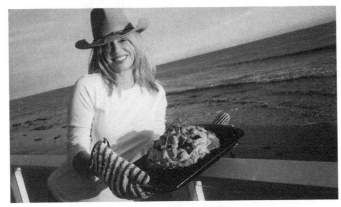

A mountain of Berry Pie with a whole wheat crust.

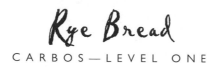

Rye Bread
CARBOS — LEVEL ONE

MAKES 1 (1½-POUND) LOAF

I love rye bread. This one is easy to make, as long as you have an automatic bread machine (available at cooking stores). Also, pick up an instant-read thermometer at a grocery store. They are inexpensive and handy to keep in the kitchen drawer. Whole wheat bread flour is best because of the high gluten content. If you can't find it, use whole wheat pastry flour.

2½ cups whole wheat bread flour
1 cup rye flour
1 tablespoon unsweetened cocoa powder
   (see Note)
1½ teaspoons caraway seeds

1 teaspoon salt
1 cup plus 2 tablespoons water
⅓ cup nonfat dried milk powder
½ cup nonfat plain yogurt
2 teaspoons active dry yeast

Mix together whole wheat bread flour, rye flour, cocoa powder, caraway seeds, and salt in a bowl. Set aside.

In a saucepan whisk together water and milk powder. Stir in the nonfat yogurt. Using an instant-read thermometer, heat the mixture to 80 degrees over low heat.

Place all the ingredients in a bread machine following the manufacturer's guidelines. Bake using the whole wheat cycle.

Note

Cocoa powder creates a minor imbalance. If you are doing well on Level One, you should be able to incorporate this small amount without creating a problem.

Multigrain Bread

MAKES 1 (1 1/2-POUND) LOAF

This bread has great texture, with rolled oats and wheat germ. As I mentioned in the other bread recipes, you will need an automatic bread maker, available at cooking stores. It's an investment, but you will love being able to enjoy totally Somersized bread in the morning. Whole wheat bread flour is best because of the high gluten content. If you can't find it, use whole wheat pastry flour.

3/4 cup rolled oats
1/4 cup toasted wheat germ
2 1/2 cups whole wheat bread flour
1 teaspoon salt

1 cup plus 2 tablespoons water
5 tablespoons nonfat dried milk powder
1/3 cup nonfat plain yogurt
2 teaspoons active dry yeast

Place rolled oats in a small nonstick skillet. Cook over medium heat, stirring occasionally until oats give off a nutty aroma and turn golden brown. Cool to room temperature and mix with the toasted wheat germ in a bowl. Set aside.

Mix together whole wheat bread flour and salt in a bowl. Set aside.

In a saucepan whisk together water and milk powder. Stir in the nonfat yogurt. Using an instant-read thermometer, heat the mixture to 80 degrees over low heat.

Place the milk mixture, flour mixture, and yeast in a bread machine, following the manufacturer's guidelines. Bake using the whole wheat cycle.

Add the toasted oats and wheat germ 5 minutes into the first knead cycle.

Tabbouleh

SERVES 4

I love the fresh taste of tabbouleh. It's a staple in the Middle Eastern diet and lucky for us, it's Somersized because it's whole-grain wheat. This takes only moments to make and is delicious served with my Middle Eastern Vegetable Stew (p. 206).

1 cup bulgur wheat
1½ cups vegetable stock
2 cloves garlic, minced
2 tablespoons lemon juice

1 scallion, chopped
¼ cup chopped fresh parsley
Salt and freshly ground black pepper

Put bulgur in a mixing bowl.

In a saucepan, heat the stock and garlic, bringing to a boil. Pour the hot stock over the bulgur. Stir, cover bowl with foil, and let bulgur stand for 30 minutes. Mix in remaining ingredients and season with salt and pepper.

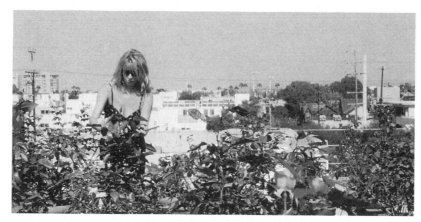

I love roses!

Hearty Mushroom Lasagna

CARBOS AND VEGGIES—LEVEL ONE

SERVES 6

You won't believe this lasagna is a Level One Carbos meal. The nonfat ricotta cheese really makes it yummy! This dish is perfect to make on Sunday afternoon and eat all week long. It's even better the day after because the flavors meld together.

FOR THE SAUCE

3 cups nonfat milk
3 tablespoons whole wheat flour
4 large cloves garlic, thinly sliced
1 teaspoon dried oregano
1 pound assorted mushrooms, thinly sliced
Salt and freshly ground black pepper

FOR THE LASAGNA ASSEMBLY

8 ounces whole wheat lasagna noodles
1 (16-ounce) can crushed tomatoes
1 pound nonfat ricotta cheese
3 tablespoons chopped fresh basil leaves
2 medium zucchini, cut in rounds
2 teaspoons chopped fresh parsley

Preheat oven to 350 degrees. Bring a large pot of salted water to a boil.

In a 4-quart saucepan, combine milk, flour, garlic, and oregano. Over medium heat, bring to a boil, stirring constantly. Add mushrooms and turn down heat to a low boil. Cook for 45 minutes or until the milk thickens into a rich sauce. Season with salt and pepper. Set aside.

When the water is boiling, add noodles and cook for about 10 minutes, just until soft. Lay out noodles on a sheet pan covered with parchment paper and set aside.

Mix together tomatoes, ricotta, and basil in a small mixing bowl.

In the bottom of an 8-inch square glass baking dish, spread one third of the tomato-cheese mixture. Lay three lasagna noodles on top of the sauce. Spread 1 cup of the mushroom sauce and layer half of the sliced zucchini. Top with another one third of the tomato-cheese mixture. Repeat lasagna noodles, mushroom sauce, and zucchini until finished. Top with remaining tomato mixture, sprinkle with chopped parsley, and bake for about 1 hour.

For Level Two
Add 1 cup Parmesan cheese to the ricotta and basil mixture.

Whole-Grain Pasta Primavera

LEVEL TWO

SERVES 4

I have come to prefer the taste of whole-grain pasta to white pasta. You can find several varieties in health food stores, such as whole wheat, spelt, amaranth, and kamut. In this Level Two recipe I toss the pasta with fresh vegetables and a little Parmesan. For Level One you would omit the oil and cheese.

2 zucchini
2 yellow squash
1 red bell pepper
1 yellow bell pepper
2 pounds snap peas
3 tablespoons olive oil

4 cloves garlic, minced
1 pound whole-grain pasta
Salt and freshly ground black pepper
2 bunches Italian parsley, chopped
Freshly grated Parmesan cheese

Place a large pot of salted water over high heat and bring to a boil.

Slice the zucchini, yellow squash, red pepper, yellow pepper, and snap peas into julienne strips of similar size. Heat a large skillet on medium heat. Add the olive oil to cover the bottom of the skillet. Add the garlic and cook until golden, about 1–2 minutes. Turn the heat to high and add the vegetables,

sautéing until just tender, about 4–5 minutes.

Add the pasta to the boiling water and cook as per the package instructions. Drain in a colander and place pasta in a bowl. Add the sautéed vegetables. Toss everything together and liberally salt and pepper. Add more olive oil, if necessary, to coat all the pasta. Sprinkle with chopped Italian parsley and Parmesan cheese.

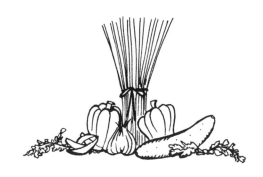

Vegetables and Side Dishes

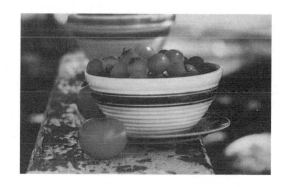

Green Chili Celery Root Puree

PRO/FATS AND VEGGIES—LEVEL ONE

SERVES 6

Each of my Somersize books has had a different recipe for celery root puree. You think I like the stuff? It's the perfect substitute for mashed potatoes. This version is spiced up with green chilies for my Southwest Christmas. If you don't want to roast your own chilies, use canned Ortega chilies.

6 fresh pasilla chilies (or 8 ounces canned
   Ortega chilies)
3 celery roots

¼ cup heavy cream
4 tablespoons butter
Salt and freshly ground black pepper

Roast the chilies over a hot grill or over a gas burner. Turn them until the skin is bubbling and charred on all sides. Place the chilies in a plastic bag for about 15 minutes. To remove the skin, take the chilies out of the bag and peel off the blackened skin. Break open each chili and remove the seeds until you have only skinless strips of chili flesh.

Place about 5 cups of water in a large pot fitted with a steamer and a lid. Bring to a boil.

Chop off the roots and peel off the out-side layer of skin from the celery roots, being careful to remove all the brown. Cut each celery root into about 12 pieces, and place in the steamer. Steam until very soft when poked with a fork, about 20 minutes.

Transfer the celery root to a food processor. Add the chilies, cream, and butter, and puree until smooth. (If you don't have a food processor, you can use an electric mixer.) Add additional cream or butter to achieve desired consistency. Sprinkle with salt and pepper to taste.

Grilled Vegetable Antipasto

PRO/FATS AND VEGGIES—LEVEL ONE

SERVES 8

This platter is a colorful addition to any buffet when I'm throwing a party for my family and friends. When you quarter the radicchio and onions, leave the cores attached so they don't fall apart on the grill.

½ cup extra-virgin olive oil
2 heads radicchio, quartered
2 bulbs fennel, thinly sliced
3 red bell peppers, seeded and cut into chunky strips
1 large eggplant, sliced into ½-inch rounds
1 pound baby onions
2 red onions, quartered

8 long sprigs fresh rosemary
Salt and freshly ground black pepper
8 Candied Tomatoes (from *Eat Great, Lose Weight*, p. 76)
8 heads Baked Garlic (from *Eat Great, Lose Weight*, p. 80)
8 lemon wedges
A drizzle of balsamic vinegar for garnish

Preheat the grill or grill pan.

Pour the olive oil into a large mixing bowl. Toss the prepared radicchio, fennel, bell peppers, eggplant, baby onions, red onions, and rosemary in the olive oil and season with salt and pepper. Place them on the hot grill, turning several times and removing once black grill marks have appeared. The vegetables are best-tasting when they are tender but still slightly crisp. Arrange them on a platter until all are cooked.

Roughly chop the candied tomatoes and add to the platter. Squeeze the cloves of baked garlic into a small bowl, then spread evenly over the vegetables. Drizzle with lemon and balsamic vinegar.

Rosemary-Infused Savory Custard with Tomato Mushroom Sauce

PRO/FATS AND VEGGIES—LEVEL ONE

SERVES 6

The French love custards. In America we think of custard as a dessert, as in crème caramel or flan. This custard is a beautiful accompaniment to roast leg of lamb or any roasted or braised meat. It is delicious with all sorts of sauces, but I particularly like this tomato mushroom sauce. It can be a meal on its own (perfect for vegetarians) or with a strong meat flavor. Make this early in the day so there is not so much work at mealtime.

3 cups heavy cream
1 cup water
6 tablespoons minced fresh rosemary
4 bay leaves
4 eggs
2 egg yolks
1/4 cup freshly grated Parmesan cheese
1/4 teaspoon freshly grated nutmeg

1/4 teaspoon sea salt
Freshly ground black pepper
1 recipe Tomato Mushroom Sauce (p. 193)
1 sprig rosemary for garnish

EQUIPMENT

6 1-cup ramekins

Preheat oven to 350 degrees.

Butter 6 1-cup ramekins.

In a medium-size saucepan, combine cream, water, rosemary, and bay leaves, and scald over high heat, bringing the mixture just to the boiling point. Remove from heat, and allow to cool. Strain the liquid through a fine-mesh sieve into a large bowl. Discard herbs.

In a small bowl blend eggs and egg yolks lightly with a fork. (Don't let the mixture get foamy or frothy or the custard will be filled with bubbles.)

When the cream mixture has cooled, add eggs and stir to blend. Stir in cheese, nutmeg, salt, and pepper. Taste for seasoning.

Divide custard among ramekins and place the ramekins in a roasting pan. Add enough hot water to roasting pan to reach halfway up the sides of the ramekins. Place in center of oven and bake about 50–55 minutes, until the custards are just set at the edges but still soft in the center. Remove from water bath and invert onto serving dish. Spoon Tomato Mushroom Sauce around the edges and garnish with sprig of rosemary.

Tomato Mushroom Sauce

PRO/FATS AND VEGGIES—LEVEL ONE

SERVES 6

This is a delicious sauce for my Rosemary-Infused Savory Custard (p. 192). You may also try it on whole wheat pasta, but because of the olive oil, save that combination for Level Two.

¼ cup extra-virgin olive oil
1 small onion, minced
3 cloves garlic, minced
1 stalk celery, minced
Salt
8 ounces mushrooms, thinly sliced (shiitake, cremini, portobello, or regular button mushrooms)

1 (28-ounce) can crushed Italian plum tomatoes with juice
1 teaspoon chopped fresh Italian parsley
1 bay leaf
Freshly ground black pepper

Combine oil, onion, garlic, celery, and a sprinkle of salt in a medium saucepan. Cook on medium low heat for about 5 minutes, until vegetables are soft.

Add the mushrooms and sauté until the mushrooms are browned and a little crusty, about 10 minutes. Add the crushed tomatoes and their juice, the parsley, and bay leaf and turn up the heat to medium. Simmer, uncovered, about 15 minutes, until sauce begins to thicken.

Season with salt and pepper to taste.

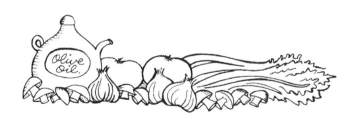

Grilled Artichokes

PRO/FATS AND VEGGIES—LEVEL ONE

SERVES 2

I'm always looking for new ways to prepare artichokes. These are grilled with a little wine and garlic, then served with delicious Green Goddess Dressing.

2 large artichokes
1 lemon, halved
4 tablespoons olive oil
4 tablespoons white wine (see Note)
4 cloves garlic, chopped

Salt and freshly ground black pepper
1 recipe Green Goddess Dressing (p. 149)
 or melted butter or mayonnaise for
 dipping

Preheat a grill or grill pan.

Using kitchen scissors, remove the sharp tips from the artichoke leaves. With a knife, cut off stems, then cut the artichokes in half lengthwise. Rub all sides of the artichokes with lemon. Brush each artichoke, on both sides, with a tablespoon of olive oil. Place on hot grill for 5 minutes, slightly charring both sides. Remove and place each half, cut side down, in the center of a piece of foil (approximately 12 inches square). Pour 1 tablespoon of wine over each artichoke. Sprinkle with chopped garlic, salt, and pepper.

Gather the four corners of each foil sheet together and twist to close. Place back on grill for about 1 hour. Carefully remove the foil, allowing the steam to escape. Remove the choke with a sharp knife.

Dip the leaves in Green Goddess Dressing, melted butter, or mayonnaise.

Note

If you are doing well on Level One, this modest amount of wine should not cause a problem.

Asparagus with Butter and Parmesan

PRO/FATS AND VEGGIES—LEVEL ONE

SERVES 4

Asparagus is one of my favorite vegetables, and it's so healthy for you. You'll love it with this burned butter and Parmesan.

2 tablespoons salt
1 pound asparagus, washed and tough
   lower stems removed

2 tablespoons butter
1 tablespoon extra-virgin olive oil
½ cup freshly grated Parmesan cheese

Prepare an "ice bath" of a large bowl filled with ice water and set aside. Bring a large pot of water to a boil and add the salt. Add the asparagus and cook until tender but still a little crunchy, about 8 minutes. Remove the asparagus and immediately plunge into the ice bath to stop the cooking process. Drain the asparagus as soon as it is cool. Don't let it sit in the water too long or it will get mushy.

Heat a large skillet over medium heat and add butter and oil. Let the butter and oil get nice and hot, then add the asparagus. Sauté just until heated through, about 2–3 minutes. Transfer the asparagus to a platter, sprinkle with cheese, and serve immediately.

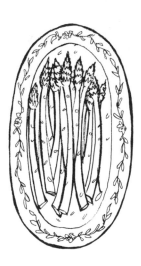

Caramelized Fennel

SERVES 4

This slow-cooked fennel gets sweet and golden. It's the perfect side dish for my Rosemary Roast Loin of Pork (p. 229). What a dinner!

4 large fennel bulbs, trimmed and thinly
  sliced
2 tablespoons extra-virgin olive oil

2 tablespoons butter
Salt and freshly ground black pepper

Place the fennel in a bowl and toss with olive oil. Heat a large skillet over medium high heat and melt the butter. Add the fennel and reduce heat to low. Continue cooking for about 1 hour, stirring occasionally. The fennel will become soft and caramelized to a beautiful golden brown. Season with salt and pepper.

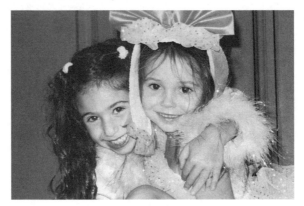

*Our granddaughters dressed as poodles
before a ballet recital.*

Fennel with Butter and Parmesan Cheese

PRO/FATS AND VEGGIES—LEVEL ONE

SERVES 6

Every year I wait for fennel to come into season. It is one of those vegetables that is delicious raw and sliced in salads, or cooked to a soft, yummy tenderness. I am always looking for something to serve that gives the feeling that you are having a potato course (or carbohydrate), without actually cheating. This satisfies the potato cravings better than anything I know.

Salt
8 small fennel bulbs, trimmed and
  quartered

5 tablespoons butter
Salt and freshly ground black pepper
1 cup freshly grated Parmesan cheese

Heat the broiler.

Bring a large pot of salted water to a boil over high heat. Add the quartered fennel bulbs and cook until slightly softened, about 5 minutes. Drain and set aside.

Heat a large skillet over medium heat. Add butter and swirl in pan until melted. Add fennel and season to taste with salt and pepper. Cook until just tender, about 5 minutes, turning occasionally.

Transfer to a casserole dish and sprinkle with Parmesan cheese. Place under the broiler for 1–2 minutes, or until cheese is golden and bubbly. Serve immediately.

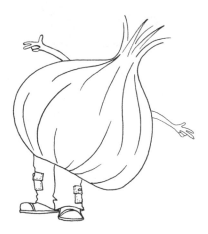

Chinese Long Beans

SERVES 4 – 6

Chinese long beans have a beautiful, festive look. Try tying them in bundles for an elegant presentation.

1 pound Chinese long beans
4 tablespoons peanut oil
1 tablespoon grated fresh ginger

3 tablespoons soy sauce
Juice of 1 lemon
Freshly ground black pepper

Trim the ends off the long beans.

Heat a large sauté pan over high heat. Add 3 tablespoons of the peanut oil, then the long beans, and cook until tender, about 5 minutes. Remove the long beans and set aside on a platter.

In the same pan, reduce the heat to low and add the last tablespoon of peanut oil and the ginger. Sauté until golden, about 3 minutes. Add the soy sauce, lemon juice, and pepper. Pour the sauce over the long beans and serve.

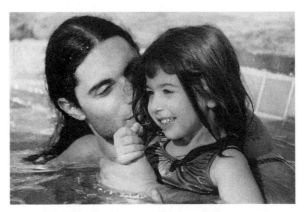

Frank with his daughter.

Gingered Snap Peas

SERVES 4

So many people say they don't like vegetables. That's because they've only eaten bland frozen or canned veggies that have been overcooked. People tell me they eat more vegetables than ever because my recipes make them taste so good. These snap peas are paired with ginger, soy, and a kick of cayenne.

¼ cup peanut oil
3 tablespoons finely chopped fresh ginger
3 cloves garlic, minced
1 pound snap peas

2 tablespoons soy sauce
¼ teaspoon cayenne pepper
Salt and freshly ground black pepper

Heat oil in a sauté pan. Add the ginger and garlic. Cook for about 3 minutes, until both are golden brown. Add the snap peas and sauté, stirring constantly, for 1 minute. Add the soy sauce and continue cooking for 1 additional minute. Add cayenne pepper, stir, and transfer to a bowl. Toss peas and let stand, loosely covered, for 5 minutes. Season with salt and pepper and serve.

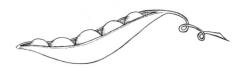

Portobello Mushrooms with Bubbling Pesto

PRO/FATS AND VEGGIES—LEVEL ONE

SERVES 4

These mushrooms make a great appetizer or a delicious accompaniment for a summer meal alongside a steak. They work especially well if you are using your outdoor grill, but you can also broil them in the oven.

4 large portobello mushrooms
Olive oil for brushing
Salt and freshly ground black pepper

1 recipe Basil Pesto (p. 155)
4 tablespoons freshly grated Parmesan
  cheese

Trim the stems off the mushrooms. Brush mushrooms with olive oil and season lightly. Cook gill side down over medium coals or in the broiler for 5 minutes.

Turn the mushrooms over and spread a spoonful of pesto over the entire surface. Continue to cook for 10 minutes or until the mushrooms are very tender and the pesto is bubbling. Sprinkle the Parmesan on top of the pesto and return to broiler until cheese is melted and golden.

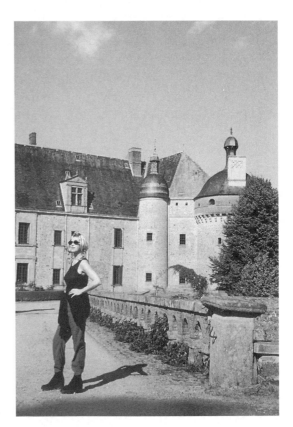

Summers spent at Jean Pierre's chateau.

Sautéed Spinach with Garlic, Lemon, and Oil

PRO/FATS AND VEGGIES—LEVEL ONE

SERVES 4

This spinach makes a great side dish for meat, poultry, or fish. I love garlic, lemon, and olive oil on just about anything; it really brings spinach to life.

2 tablespoons salt
2 pounds fresh spinach, rinsed and
    destemmed
2 tablespoons extra-virgin olive oil

4 cloves garlic, thinly sliced
Salt and freshly ground black pepper
Juice from 1 lemon

Bring a large pot of water to a boil over high heat. Add the salt and the spinach, stirring until the spinach is just wilted, about 2 minutes. Drain the spinach and rinse thoroughly with cold water. Drain well, pressing as much liquid out of the spinach as possible.

Transfer spinach to a chopping block and coarsely chop. Heat a large skillet over medium heat, then add the olive oil and garlic. Saute the garlic for 1–2 minutes until golden. Add the chopped spinach and gently toss with the garlic until heated through, about 2–3 minutes. Season with salt, pepper, and the lemon juice. Serve immediately.

Spicy Broccoli

SERVES 4

Add a little heat to your broccoli and it's like a whole new vegetable. Alan and I eat this for dinner and then dance around the living room, salsa style. We like it hot!

¼ cup peanut oil
2 teaspoons toasted sesame oil
6 cloves garlic, minced

1 pound broccoli florets, blanched
2 teaspoons soy sauce
1 teaspoon dried red pepper flakes

Heat both oils in a large skillet. Add the garlic and sauté for 1–2 minutes or until golden brown. Add the broccoli and cook for about 5 minutes, until it is tender but still a little crunchy. Add the soy sauce and continue to cook for 1 minute. Toss to coat the broccoli. Stir in the red pepper flakes and serve.

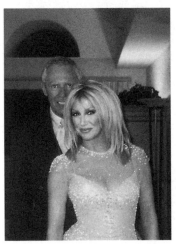

Alan and me—a night out in Hollywood.

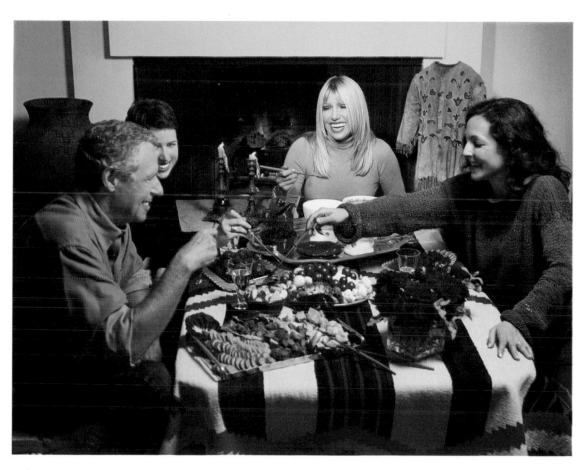

A fondue party can be a fun way to spend time with friends and family. Here we have Swiss Cheese Fondue, Meat Fondue, bubbling broth, and vegetables for dipping.

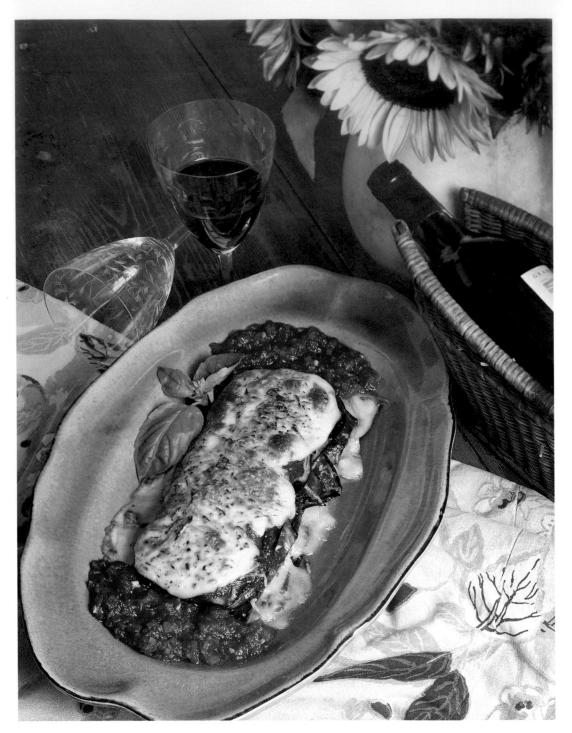

Eggplant Parmesan

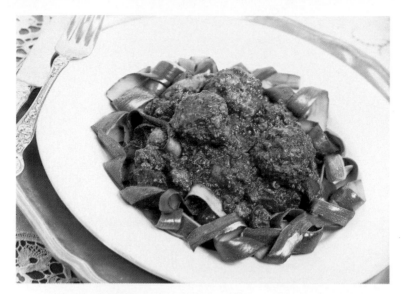

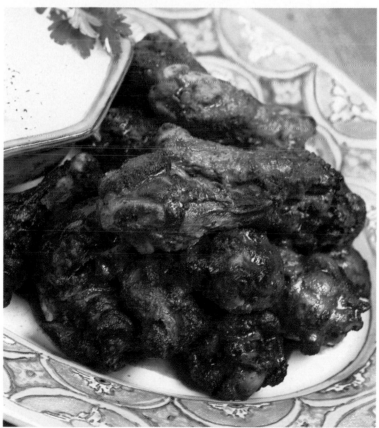

TOP: Meatballs and Zucchini Noodles
BOTTOM: Buffalo Wings with Blue Cheese Dip

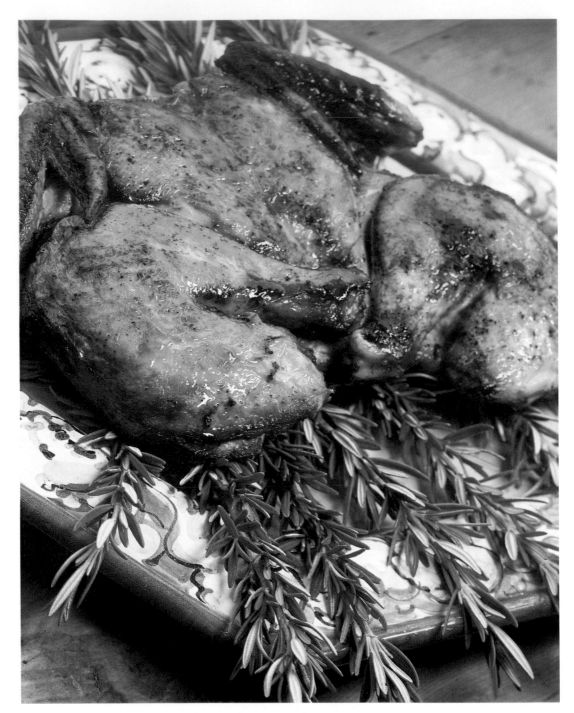

Flattened Chicken

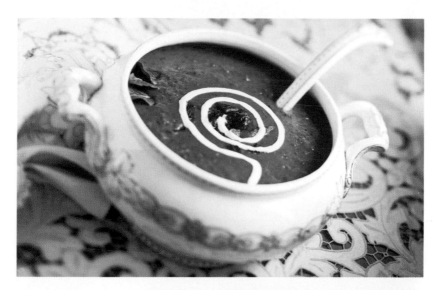

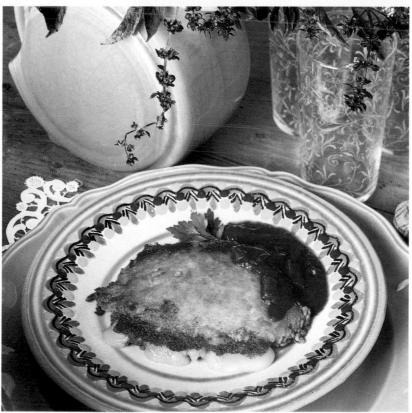

TOP: Roasted Sweet Red Pepper Soup with Crème Fraîche and Crispy Sage Leaves
BOTTOM: Mozzarella Marinara

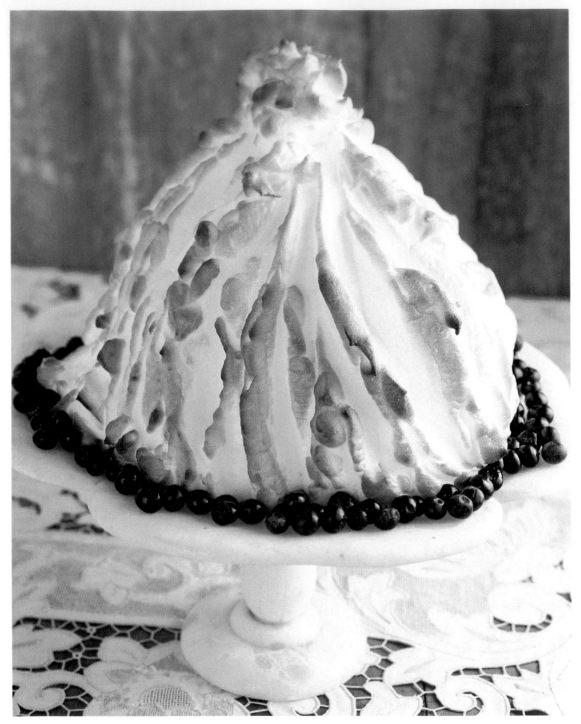

Black-and-White Baked Alaska